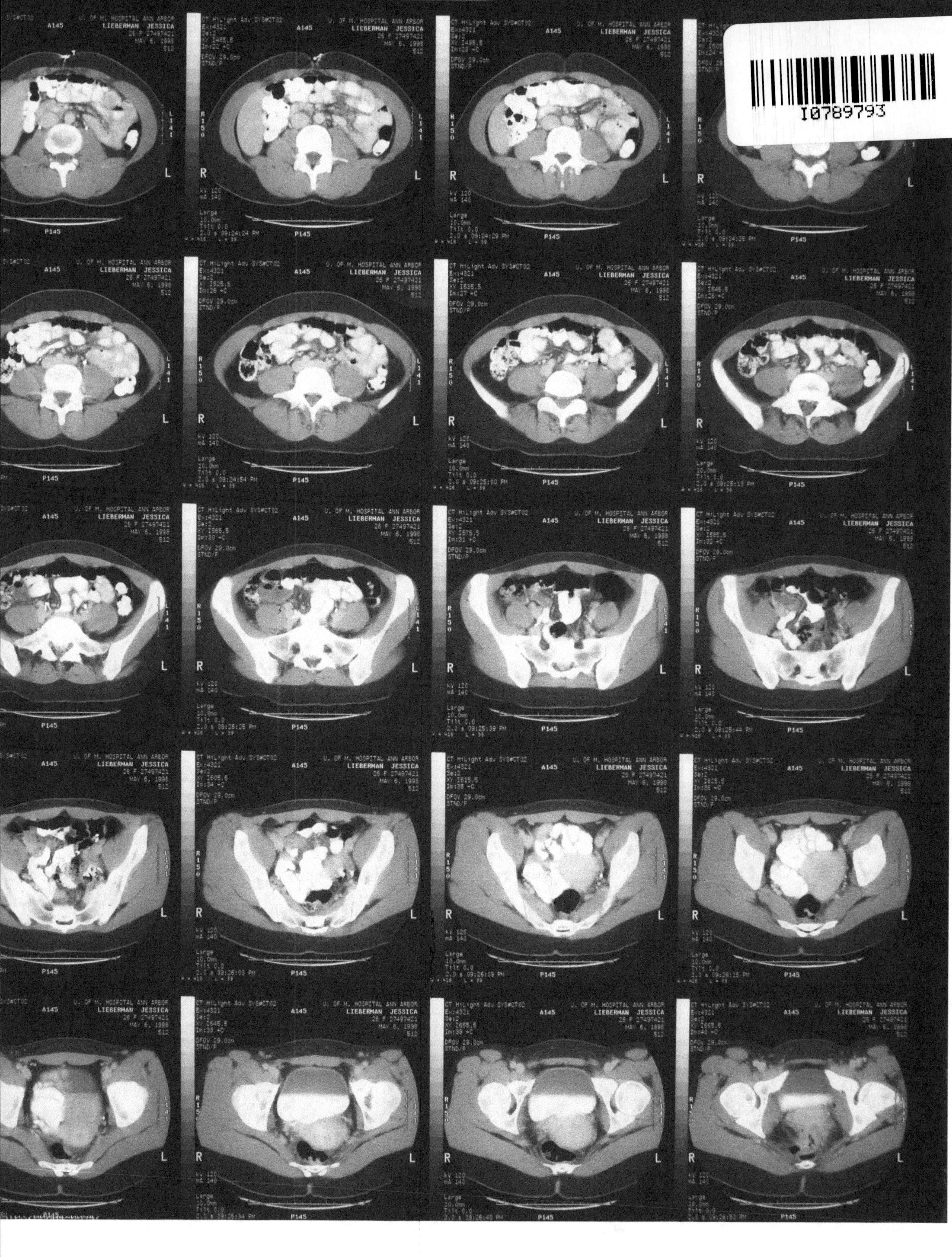

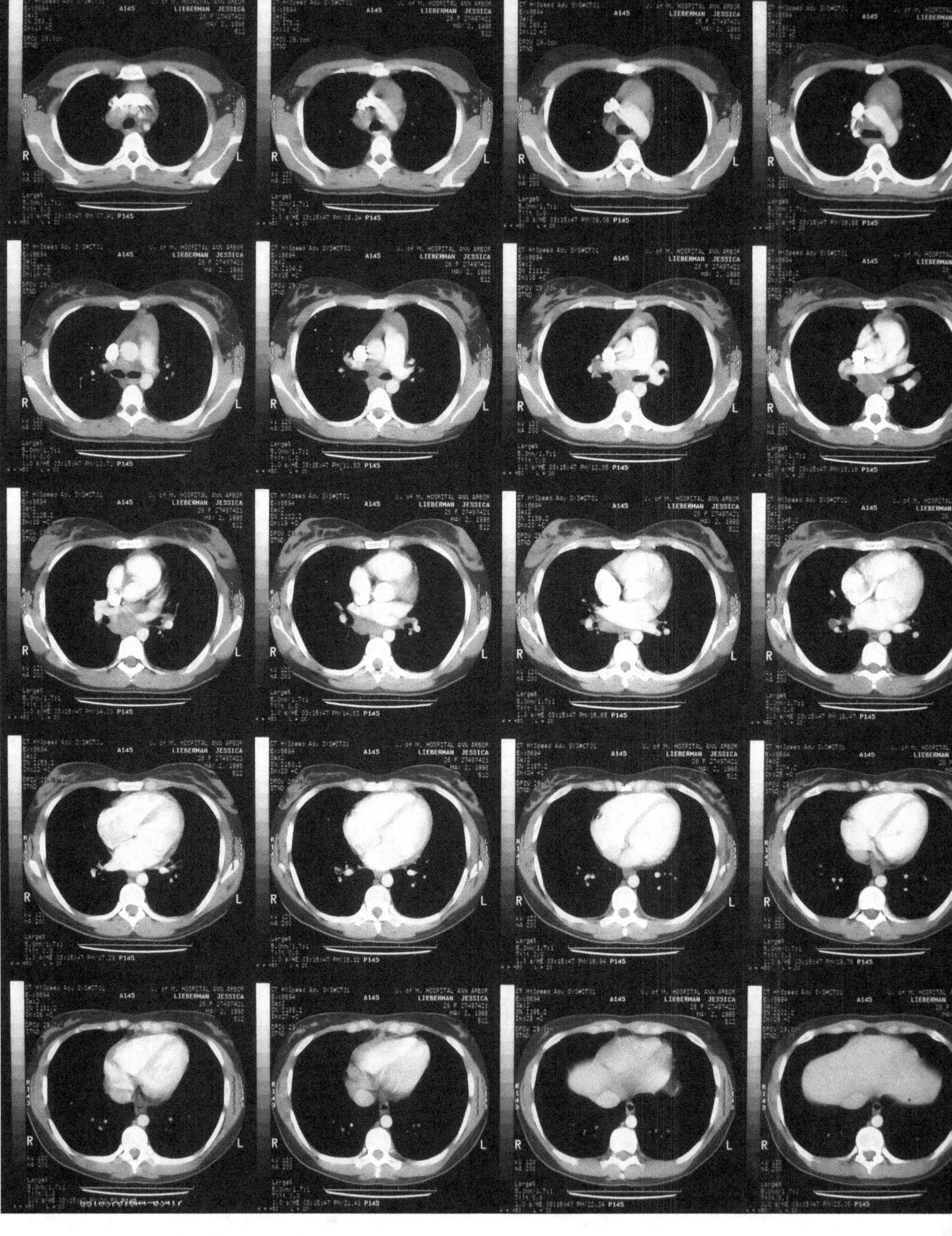

BECOMING VISIBLE

BECOMING VISIBLE

JESSICA CATHERINE LIEBERMAN

RIT PRESS
ROCHESTER, NY

Becoming Visible

© 2013 Rochester Institute of Technology and Jessica Lieberman
All rights reserved. No part of this book may be used or reproduced
in any manner without written permission.

RIT Press
90 Lomb Memorial Drive
Rochester, New York 14623-5604
http://ritpress.rit.edu

Book and cover design by Marnie Soom
Printed in the U.S.A.

Library of Congress Cataloging-in-Publication Data

Lieberman, Jessica Catherine, 1971–
    Becoming visible / Jessica Catherine Lieberman.
       pages   cm
    ISBN 978-1-933360-82-9 (alk. paper) — ISBN 97801933360836 (e-book)
    1. Lieberman, Jessica Catherine, 1971—Health. 2. Lieberman, Jessica
Catherine, 1971—Self-portraits. 3. Hodgkin's disease–Patients–Biography–
Pictorial works. I. Title.
    RC644.L54 2013
    616.99'4460092–dc23
    [B]
                                                        2013030894

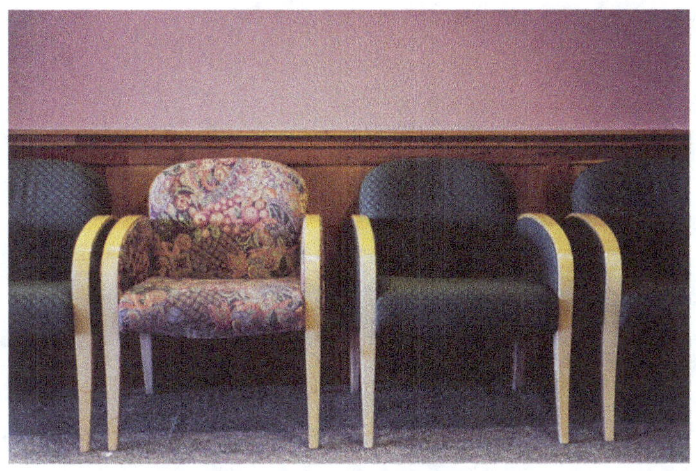

For Amit, who handled it all.

CONTENTS

Foreword

Albert J. Winn

Illness is debilitating, destabilizing. I'm not referring to a
cold, which is uncomfortable, or the flu, which can knock
your socks off for a while, but a real, genuinely frightening,
life-threatening disease. One debases and dehumanizes you
in the most unimaginable ways. A disease that takes on a
life of its own, seems to reach out from some unexpected
place, sucks you in and swallows until you and the disease
are one. It steals your identity in such a way that if you
were standing in line waiting to hear your name called, you
wouldn't recognize the sound, the pronunciation, the spell-
ing. When you look in the mirror, you are unrecognizable.
"That's not me. That's someone else," you hear yourself
screaming inside your head. You are now a prisoner in a
foreign land, in an alien culture with a language, a nomen-
clature, you don't understand. You are poked and prodded;
substances are injected and extracted. There are rules,
regulations, protocols to follow, people to whom you can't
speak, people who dictate your actions and your speech.
It feels as if you are in an environment that has rendered
you invisible.

Your struggle is to survive even when you know the odds
are long. Your struggle is to push back even when it seems
that you are being enveloped by a cloud. Your struggle is

to get the vocabulary, the syntax straight, so that you can
understand, so that you can speak and be heard. Your
struggle is to shake up the very people who say they are
trying to save your life, to make them see you, and for you,
now dependent on them, not to forget who you are, that
you were once a self-sufficient being. You want to somehow
show your humanity, so that even if you die, all you really
want to know is that you were seen. And even if you recover,
you always remember, live with just a trace of fear, that your
life could get sucked back up again.

I know what this is. I have traveled this route, although
mine was AIDS before there was an effective treatment. I
was told that little could be done and to prepare to waste
away. Support groups were useless. Like Jessica Lieberman,
I sneaked a camera into the hospital to make similar pictures of my treatments, experienced the same bureaucratic
systems that seemed to separate me from my own body,
desperately sought out drug protocols, was asked the same
astounding questions from the well, the uninfected, the yet
to be diagnosed who thought that we, the diseased, who
know our life will end, have an insightfulness about life's
mysteries. I worried that my illness was taxing my spouse,
wearing him down. I could recognize those who carried
the same illness and what they were experiencing merely
by their physiognomy. It revealed their secrets. It was our
fraternal handshake. No matter the seriousness of the
tale, this book made me remember those dark days, made
me remember the fear, compelled me to re-examine the pictures. It made me laugh out loud.

Photographs and stories do not just stand alone. Whether
we want them to or not, they compel us into a narrative of
our own making, allow us to insert something of ourselves
into the image, the story. For all of us who have experienced
this foreign land, these tales, these photographs, the discourse in Jessica Lieberman's book will seem autobiograph-
ical. The photographs here are what the patient sees. A
treatment room that could be an execution chamber, a bald
head that references a prisoner and chemotherapy. They

tell us how profoundly uncomfortable the diagnosed, the
ill, the person in treatment feels. For all those who may one
day follow, for all those who just want to know, and all those
who should know about the world of being ill, *Becoming
Visible* lets us in, makes it clear.

Albert J. Winn
Photographer

Stealing Images of Herself

Therese Mulligan

In 1998, writer and image-maker Jessica Lieberman began life-saving treatment for Hodgkin's lymphoma. For two years, she endured the labyrinthine construct of the American health system, moving through hospital waiting rooms and cancer centers for inpatient and outpatient care. Assembled teams of doctors, nurses, and technicians charted every minute step of her treatment in files that systematically documented in word and image patient observations and administration of therapies. Along the way, Lieberman compiled her own dossier of her experience of living with cancer, including the all too human side of medical care, with its dire accompaniment of physical and mental suffering. To capture her experience, she smuggled cameras into hospital rooms, often hidden in the voluminous folds of blankets that kept her warm as she healed from surgery or received her next round of chemotherapy. Although hospital regulations banned the use of personal cameras, Lieberman decided to "steal" images of herself, knowing that, as she writes in her essay here, "I could worry less about the days and weeks that were passing me by if I felt that a record was being kept."

Becoming Visible is much more than a therapeutic picture book with text of one individual's journey of living with and then surviving a life-threatening disease. It is a first-person study that examines the philosophical underpinning of visual representation when the subject depicted involves personal trauma and its associated social import. As a theorist and academician whose scholarly work takes up themes from visual culture, Lieberman importantly combines resonant views from cultural studies, critical theory, and philosophy in her introductory essay to underscore the social relevance of seeing and describing, looking at and interpreting the picturing of the self via the photographic record. She draws upon those writers whose influence has done much to condition our contemporary understanding of photography: Roland Barthes, Susan Sontag, Carol Squiers, and Hervé Guibert, to name but a few. Significantly, in *Becoming Visible*, Lieberman also engages in and adds to the growing literature of trauma studies, a field for which photography holds great consequence with its inextricable ties to evidence, memory, and the politics and economies of visual representation.

In *Becoming Visible*, Lieberman astutely interweaves a diaristic mode of storytelling with blunt and candid snapshot photographs, medical documents, and body scans. Text and image build upon one another, creating an intricate visual story of personal pathography, an intense examination of a life lived under constant threat of disease. This monograph serves, on the one hand, as a means for Lieberman to remember and contemplate her own pictorial and written interventions into her experience with cancer. On the other, its scope is much greater. It looks to posit connections with the future survivor-self and with new audiences, who view these pages or encounter the stolen images laid out on gallery walls, by making publicly visible the profound and often unseen effects of illness.

Therese Mulligan. Ph.D.
Chair, School of Photographic Arts and Sciences
and Gallery Director

Becoming Visible

IF ONE IS TO BECOME VISIBLE, the question is—or so it seems to me now, many years later—whom is one becoming visible to? Who is to be the new viewer, the witness? Who will be made to "see" something previously unseen, something unseeable? When I first decided to show the images and writing I had produced while undergoing treatment for Hodgkin's lymphoma, I realized that I would not simply be sharing something personal, but would also be engaging in a politics of representation: revealing unseen suffering by rhetorically and visually constituting a complex system of social practices, medical conventions, discursive patterns, personal anecdotes, and iconic motifs in order to bear witness, give testimony, substantiate. In March of 2000, I installed thirty-two color photographs, interwoven in series with seven works of written text, on the walls of the gallery in Angell Hall at the University of Michigan. Titled "Becoming Visible," the exhibition was inspired by my experiences of the prior two years with diagnosis, surgery, chemotherapy, radiation, and recovery.

Although the complex politics of objectification was a factor in my choices, the question of audience was not one I was concerned with during treatment. Indeed, the only person I was trying to reach, to commune with, to show something to, was myself. That was very clear to me at the time. The photographs were for me, the writing was for me—not necessarily as therapeutic processes, but as communications from the present to the future. This was an important distinction. I wanted to reveal my current state to a potential future self, a "survivor," a self that might just "move on" from this experience and no longer be the cancer-self I felt myself to have become. These words, these images, these traces were meant to embody a time in my life, and a self in my life, that was not visible to me. At the same time, writing and photographing were an avoidance. Roland Barthes famously quotes Franz Kafka as responding to a provocation that sight is the "necessary condition" for an image. Kafka, he explains, "smiled and replied: 'We photograph things in order to *drive them out* of our minds. My stories are a way of *shutting* my eyes'" (Barthes 1981, 53, emphases mine). I could worry less about the days and weeks that were passing me by if I felt that a record was being kept. I could simultaneously distance myself from my own discomfort if I "captured" my experience photographically and, therefore, need not process it as it would be available, if needed, to consider later.

A therapeutic distance and means of control produced by the mediating lens of the camera: this is a provocative concept. Susan Sontag spent a career exploring the question of a photograph's ability to evidence events at the same time that it provides distance from the experience for a viewer. A photograph, she argues, "is not only like its subject, a homage to the subject. It is part of, an extension of that subject; and a potent means of acquiring it, of gaining control over it" (Sontag 1978, 155). Photographic documentation is a way to confirm "that the subject exists" (165), and a way of "imprisoning reality, understood as recalcitrant, inaccessible; of making it stand still" (163). My camera could provide a means to insist upon my own subjective viewpoint, to exert control over my reality, and, further still, to create a sense of a future, a survival: "Cameras establish an inferential relation to the present . . . [and] provide an instantly retroactive view of experience" (167). The downside to these exertions, however, is profound. In her earlier writings, Sontag is highly skeptical about the hope for "free political choice" in an "image-world": "Social change is replaced by a change in images . . . Cameras are the antidote and the disease, a means of appropriating reality and a means of making it obsolete" (178-79). Further still, Sontag's work anchors numerous critical discussions of the problems of desensitization to disturbing images and inurement to the pain of others that now proliferate in academic and popular media circles. The difference in my work at that time, however, is that I was capturing the images *of myself*, for my own viewing. Questions of audience reception and circulation, questions of making a spectacle out of my own pain—these were not yet on my radar. More to the point for me was the argument of photographer and philosopher Hervé Guibert—who used photography and video to document his own illness and death—who claimed that it is necessary to "live things first" before imaging them so that they don't remain "misunderstood, unlived" (Guibert 1991). This was both the potential and the danger of making these images. In trying to provide an opportunity to become visible to myself in the future, would I be avoiding or blocking my experience in the present?

Such photographic interventions into reality were stymied, however, as hospital staff informed me that photography was not permitted inside any of the cancer center buildings. I did not expect to make images of other people's private suffering. But I was surprised that I could not photograph myself, my surroundings, my personal experience. Notably, I originally learned of the ban when I was trying to access copies of the seemingly endless diagnostic images that were being made of me. This was before the enactment of the new HIPPA laws but well after the digital overhaul of testing equipment. It would be easy to e-mail an image file of my CT scans or MRIs. It would take seconds to copy my X-rays and sonograms to a disc. But I was not permitted to have copies of the images made of my own body by my medical team. As a patient, it appeared, I did not have a right to my own image. Faced with this frustration, I felt that with every new image my doctors and technicians made of me, I was becoming, in effect, less visible to myself. A visual construction of my new reality as a sick

or dying person was being pieced together, but I could not
see it. And it was a very important construction: it determined my treatment plan, how I would live the following
year, whether I would survive. Large red *x*'s marked sites
of abnormality, of danger, of difference on pictures of my
insides. Images existed, images that defined me, but they
were not mine and I had no control over them; so I simply
began to make my own images, to photograph what I saw
and to photograph myself.

I stole images of myself and my experience. Small digital
cameras and camera phones were not yet on the radar, so
I assembled a team of plastic Holga cameras, along with
my Pentax K1000 and any film I had lying around from
other projects. Because I was not experiencing temperature
in normal ways and was cold all the time, my time in the
cancer center was spent in oversized coats that happened
to have multiple, large pockets—perfect for harboring
contraband cameras. Beginning in the ninety-degree heat
and sweltering humidity of late spring and early summer, I
faced my treatment routine with my army of cameras, furtively stealing awkward glimpses of my reality. These acts
of image-making felt like acts of defiance, performances
of health, a subversive insistence on living, on being in
control. Shortly before her own death of cancer—a death
that would itself be documented and published by her
photographer partner, Annie Leibovitz (2006)—Sontag
appended her formative work on photography, pain, and
cultural attitudes toward illness to celebrate the political
potential of the "unstoppable" proliferation of images of
suffering. She explains: "Photographs have an insuperable
power to determine what we recall of events . . . To live is
to be photographed, to have a record of one's life . . . But to
live is also to pose. To act is to share in the community of
actions recorded as images" (Sontag 2004b). I embraced
the performative act of imaging myself and the performative act of posing as realities in which I could assert myself
as alive while working to find agency in my world.

* * *

The hazy quality of my thoughts, actions, and perceptions during treatment was peculiar, and it shows in the images. At times, I felt that my mind was clear, sharp even—that I was keenly aware of all that was taking place around me and was more observant than ever before. I imagined that, imbued by the illness and by proximity to "the end," I had a hyper-attentiveness that allowed me to see through the distractions and straight into the heart of human interactions. I would take these opportunities of alertness to write. But, at the same time, I knew that my memory was severely impaired. I did not recall visits from concerned out-of-town friends. I could not remember whether I had eaten and would re-initiate baths as soon as I had gotten dry. Above all, I knew that time itself was altered. For one thing, I seemed to have run out of it. Not only did there appear to be a limited number of hours left to me, but I also had very few hours available each day because I was sleeping eighteen hours on average and spending much of the rest in treatment or throwing up.

Difficulties with memory and time were not simply the product of coping with illness, however. I knew that I was heavily medicated, taking daily doses of medications categorized as "amnestics" that caused partial or total loss of memory. These drugs were intended to forestall the anxiety of treatment while limiting the very experience of that treatment in the first place. That is a motive worth pausing on, as it left me grasping for a way to hold on to my experiences. Some of these medications, such as Ativan, were primarily prescribed to minimize the anxiety of sitting through hours of chemotherapy. But my prescription was not directed simply to my time in the chemo chair. My instructions were to take the medication anytime, all the time, whenever I wished. The side effects of confusion, drowsiness, amnesia, forgetfulness, and trouble in concentrating were, according to my doctors, "bonus" effects—effects that would help mitigate the difficulty of coping with my situation. And they were right. I found so much relief in this blessed bit of escape that I feared I would become addicted to benzodiazepines. One doctor reassured me that, all things considered, addiction to Ativan would be "the least of my worries."

Relief from anxiety is one thing. Drug-induced amnesia is another. By the time I finished my treatments for cancer, I had been on a near-daily regimen of amnestic medication for twelve months. I was living a life that was carefully controlled to be not fully lived—the crisp realities of experience were smudged just enough that I recognized my routine as annoying, frustrating, and difficult, but also as hazy both in the moment and in recollection. And this was not the only amnesiac drug used in my treatment. I was also given Versed during some of my diagnostic procedures. Versed, like Ativan, makes you sleepy, relaxes you, and decreases your memory of events. Unlike its cousin, however, Versed is an intense and short-term sedative, usually used for operations and procedures in which the patient needs to be awake enough to respond to simple commands, but must also not have any recollection of what she just went through. So, although my long-term experience in cancer treatment was modified by amnestic medications, my precise experiences with these procedures on Versed were completely obliterated from memory. Furthermore, as I cannot recall them, the experiences of the procedures are ones that I know I had, but that I cannot assess, interrogate, or view. They are invisible to me now, though I know that they live on as meaningful experiences somewhere in my self. As a scholar of trauma, I am fascinated and troubled by these missing parts of my experience.

Trauma studies scholars define the pathology of trauma as just this kind of lost and haunting experience. In the highly influential book *Trauma: Explorations in Memory*, Cathy Caruth explains: "The experience of trauma, the fact of latency, would thus seem to consist, not in the forgetting of a reality that can hence never be fully known, but in an inherent latency within the experience itself. The historical power of the trauma is not just that the experience is repeated after its forgetting, but that it is only in and through its inherent forgetting that it is first experienced at all. . . . since the

traumatic event is not experienced as it occurs, it is fully ev-
ident only in connection with another place, and in another
time" (Caruth 1995, 7-8). The structure of trauma is defined
by disruptions of time and disturbances in the processes of
memory and forgetting such that an individual is left with
an *experience* of events that registers as a perpetual present.
The event cannot be digested and left behind as past. It is
a recurrent and persistent experience, forgotten in the moment lived, and then perpetually remembered in a different
way in the future. These are highly complex discussions.
The theory is intricate, and the suffering of individuals with
conditions such as post-traumatic stress disorder is significant. What I am suggesting here is that, though potentially
useful to alleviate the anxiety and stress of patients in the
moment of treatment, amnestic drugs enact a traumatic
encounter with the treatment experience, leaving patients
unable to process events as they occur, yet haunted by the
impact of those occurrences on their psyches and bodies.

It is in this traumatic register that I felt like an audience to
my own experiences. I had the sense, throughout my treatment, of experience slipping away from me. Events were
taking place, but I could not grasp them. Still more ab-
stract, I had a sense that I was having experiences that were
changing me, but that this new, developing me was being
rendered forgotten, invisible, silenced even as she was pro-
gressing. It was she whom I wanted to capture, nail down,
preserve, evidence. I wanted to document this woman and
her experiences to show something to myself as audience.

I quickly realized, however, that the compulsion to make
the photographs, to sneak, steal, and wrest control of my
own images, was only part of a larger performance of making myself visible. I needed to show the work publicly. I
had to expose the acts that felt so rebellious in an equally
dissident act of revelation. Maybe the photographs weren't
for me to view after all. The pleasure of making them was
leading to a desire to make them known, to exhibit.

It was not until I first publicly showed the work in a solo
exhibition that a whole new set of audiences became visible
to me. I sent invitations to the people I knew: academic
peers and advisors, photographer colleagues and mentors,
my doctors and friends. I imagined an audience who would
find the images and text to be clinical, scholarly, investiga-
tory. I thought they would be interested to see images that
were "stolen"—ones that I had been expressly forbidden to
take and that presumably, therefore, they were not supposed to see. I was taken aback, however, by the viewer
response. Certainly, there was reaction to a kind of exposé
quality to the work. But the revelatory aspect, as viewer
after viewer expressed, seemed to come not from revealing
the cancer center, but from my willingness to reveal my
own vision and voice. Time and again, audience members
stressed the silence and invisibility of their loved ones or
selves when coping with serious illness. Personal stories
were shared and revisited for new insights. "My sister could
never explain what it felt like to . . ." "My husband didn't
want to recount how the . . ." My daughter was only one
and did not yet have a language to express . . ."

Viewer response was emotive, insistent, ardent even. People
wanted me to know exactly who I had rendered visible for
them. The names and the stories of beloved sufferers filled
the pages of guest sign-in books I left by the door. But many
of the viewers sought me out to tell me in person what they
could now see. There were relatively few questions. There
were relatively few comments. There was a torrent of stories,
tears, and, to quote one viewer, "reclaimed experiences."

There was another audience that also caught me off guard:
my doctors. Some applied the clinical and technical gaze
that I had expected. Like my photographer colleagues and
academic advisors, they would point out details that fit our
shared experience—a detail about equipment, or spatial
layout, or a theoretical provocation. I was happy that they
did not seem to feel insulted, or targeted. After all, the show
was not an indictment—because it was not about them. But
several of my doctors reacted unexpectedly. I will mention

one that represents the point. He was a member of my
hematology team, a doctor who knew me very well. He was
in charge of my physicals, touching all parts of my body,
carefully surveying my skin, rooting around in my mouth
for sores. He had met my family, discussed sports with my
partner, shared my hometown. We spent countless hours together, discussed the weather and current events as well as
the consistency of my stool and the unlikelihood of my being able to bear children. Furthermore, he was a good man.
He was not the doctor who screwed up my meds during radiation treatment and had to covertly deliver corrected meds
to my partner in the middle of the night in an empty parking lot after I had lain unconscious in my own vomit in a
public bathroom stall. He was not the doctor who diagnosed
me with "unmarried woman's disease." Nor was he the one
who suggested that I had "graduate student syndrome." On
the contrary, this doctor was a good one. On the night of the
opening reception of my first show, I noticed as this doctor
entered the gallery and walked around. Some time later, I
saw him, looking concerned and confused, glancing at each
woman in the gallery curiously. Twice he made eye contact
with me and continued his search. When I approached him,
he asked if I could point out Jessica Lieberman to him. He
was, he explained, her doctor.

The anecdote could end there, but my doctor's response
to his mistake is the more important point. Mortified and
embarrassed, he explained he didn't recognize the present "me": with hair, eyelashes, eyebrows, and pinkness to
my skin. But he went on to interrogate his lack of recognition further. Talking to me longer, he admitted that he still
didn't know me, even looking into my eyes, hearing my
voice and mannerisms. They were familiar, but still not in-
dicative. I asked him about the images: did he recognize me
in them? He returned to the photographs and came back
some time later. He had figured it out. He knew me, of
course, but he knew me horizontal. I was a patient, lying on
my back, passive. Furthermore, he knew me in parts: skin,
eyes, mouth, heart, lungs, etc. Not as a whole. I had been a
set of horizontal parts laid bare for scrutiny. What was key

in this revelation was the doctor's own surprise and clear disappointment in his self. By not being able to identity me, he would write to me later, he had become aware of *how* he saw me and, thereby, had become visible "to himself."

I have been living with the designation of "long-term survivor" for twelve years now. Although I was driven to represent my experience during treatment, I then packed this work away. I presumed that I had simply "moved on," as the saying goes. But there is no "remission" from my cancer, and doctor's visits and diagnostic tests are regular rituals in my life. Last year, a doctor new to my case, an expert in lymphoma, told me that my treatment regimen in 1999 was "barbaric." He explained that it was only five months after the completion of my treatment that the regimen was replaced by significantly reduced medication cocktails and radiation fields. My treatment bought me time and fought off one kind of cancer. But the treatment itself is carcinogenic, and it will likely give me another form of cancer someday down the road. Radiation and chemo left me with "compromised" lungs and heart and a nonfunctioning thyroid. In conjunction with my autoimmune disorders—systemic lupus erythemotosus, Sjögren's syndrome, and Raynaud's disease—"surviving" cancer has left me with significant and daily problems with circulation, metabolism, breathing, exposure, and pain. Abetted by my continuing medications, treatment endangered my eyes, destroyed my gum tissue, and scarred my skin.

Furthermore, the experience of cancer is not over for my family or friends. There is still a halo of fragility, of potential loss, that I can glimpse upon my head when I see myself reflected in their eyes. My children, the miracle babies I was not supposed to be able to have, know that illness is a part of who mommy is. None of us understands the experience as wholly over, the cancer as cured, mommy as healthy. These reactions are complicated and in no way consistent. What all share in their variability, however, is a sense of persistence, of life courses shifted irremediably by illness and trajectoried by its presence in each new experience encountered.

10

Returning to this work now, as my own future audience, I
fear that I may disappoint my past self, and that leaves me
highly uncomfortable with this project. My goal of capturing an experience I could not fully live at the time was
achieved, in a way. There are indeed words and images that
I can visit, as a witness to my own past. And there is a text
and image project that I can share with others, so that they
can bear witness to experiences not specifically their own,
but that invoke realities they too are trying to substantiate.
These are important outcomes. There is only a very short
but highly impactful tradition of publishing books of *visual*
pathography and decidedly fewer of visual autopathography.
Scholars of the humanities have begun to study the mem-
oirs, autobiographies, biographies, and pathographies of
patients representing *their own* illness. In *Reconstructing
Illness: Studies in Pathography*, Anne Hunsaker Hawkins
provides a lengthy study of a range of pathographies, personal accounts of illness represented by the patient herself.
Susan Sontag, Arthur Frank, and Kay Toombs are notable
as scholars who produced projects that combine "the
author's perception of illness as a patient . . . blended with
the perception of illness as a literary critic or a sociologist"
(Hunsaker Hawkins 1999, xvi). Hunsaker Hawkins has
compiled an impressive and useful appendix of pathographies published in the second half of the twentieth century
and is joined by Thomas Couser, Jeffrey Aronson, and
Rachel Hall-Clifford in focusing research more specifically
on patients' stories.

A substantially smaller subset of pathography, and one
that has yet to be accounted for critically, is those stories of
personal illness created by visual artists. Using media such
as installation, drawing, painting, photography, graphic
novels, artist books, film, and video, Jo Spence, Hannah
Wilke, Catherine Lord, Martha A. Hall, Carol Chase Bjerke,
Marcia Reid Marsted, Eliot Lable, Sally Loughridge, Tom
Joslin, Derek Jarman, Hervé Guibert, Felix Gonzales Torres,
David Wojnarowicz, Albert J. Winn, Harvey Pekar, and
Marisa Acocella Marchetto are among those who document
and represent themselves living while ill. In the last two

decades, there has been much discussion in academe and the popular press of visual representations of disease, of their shock value, ubiquity, and graphic nature as well as their educational value, availability, and revelatory nature. Curators and scholars have revisited visual documentaries of bodies in pain (see especially Carol Squiers and Susan Sontag), and photographers, medical doctors, and art therapists have come together to produce numerous educational photo essays of patients in treatment. At the same time, disability studies has developed into a prominent academic field and introduced heated and divisive debate over the definitions of disability and the social models and contexts it deploys. It is an important time then, from an academic and cultural standpoint, to release to a broader audience a first-person visual study such as *Becoming Visible*. Visual accounts of life in the obscuring prism of disease are a topical and potent component of the proliferating testimonials and witness accounts of contemporary visual culture. It is crucial that these discussions include creative statements from those who would embody themselves in the discourse.

Another critical reason to visit this work now is to deploy its attempts at photographic intervention to interrogate contemporary visual economies in a now-digital era. Issues of privacy and surveillance were equally important twelve years ago, but they were of a very different character. Controls on access and distribution of medical records have been enacted at the same time that opportunities for access and distribution of images have exploded online. Circulation of images to intended and unintended audiences has dramatically increased our exposure to previously proprietary knowledge. We can find out what "cancer" looks like with great ease. Visceral, graphic, and disturbing images populate the Internet on sites ranging from educational to voyeuristic, responsible to mischievous. The images are not only easy to get, they are easy to make. High quality images can be made with small portable devices that go unnoticed in restricted settings. Today, even the most hastily made pictures are meant to be circulated and, therefore, in a digital world, will never go away. There is a permanence to image

exposure that guarantees a kind of (traumatic) recurrence.
In a 2012 symposium of scholars dedicated to articulating
the critical parameters of the study of visual culture in a
digital and global world, David Darts discussed the ways
in which practices of *hiding* have replaced the familiar
practices of seeing and looking that had occupied media
studies. In an environment so exposed to visibility, in which
all is shared as files, anonymity may be the new goal. Diana
Taylor (2012) emphasized the politics of the personal act
in this realm of visual ubiquity, discussing the need to recognize *seeing* something as also *saying* something. Acts of
hiding and exposure, of displaying the self and of witness-
ing the suffering of others on display—these are political
acts when the images are of social relevance. As Joanna
Zylinska argued in 2012, we need to shift our focus onto
the ethics of the processes of visual culture, recognizing the
activist potential of questioning how we mediate life with
visual forms and asking who and what gets imaged.

* * *

So what of the hope that my past self held, that I might one
day more fully live because I could see, in text and image,
my time with cancer? I certainly do use this archive of
stories of images to "remind" myself of experiences I have
forgotten. Much of the material comes as a surprise to me,
especially anecdotes and images I did not use in the 2000
exhibit. Of many of these glimpses into the past, I have no
memory at all. I read my own writing as if it were written
by someone else. So yes, my hyper-attentive process was
able to capture and preserve moments that my amnesiac
self was actively forgetting. I am highly grateful for access. Yet the greater function of this work may not be in
the retrieval of something lost at that time. It may be in
the act of having made those images and articulated those
thoughts. As performances of self, as interventions into my
own experience, these productions resonate as statements
of deferred experience and as connections with new audiences. My target audience at the time was a future self, the
self who writes and shoots today. And it is this current self

who, without these documents, cannot fully communicate
her experience. The loss in my experience, the gaps in my
memory—these elisions contribute to the larger, public
invisibility of illness. The process of finding new audiences,
connecting with new viewers, and speaking to new read-
ers as acts of embodied speech may be the retrieval I had
hoped for. Perhaps it is in and through others' experience
with the work that I am becoming visible to myself. It may
be that the most significant outcome, the one my cancer-
self would have appreciated above all else, is that, with camera and pen in hand, I lived to become a future audience
who would now critique my own methods and assumptions.

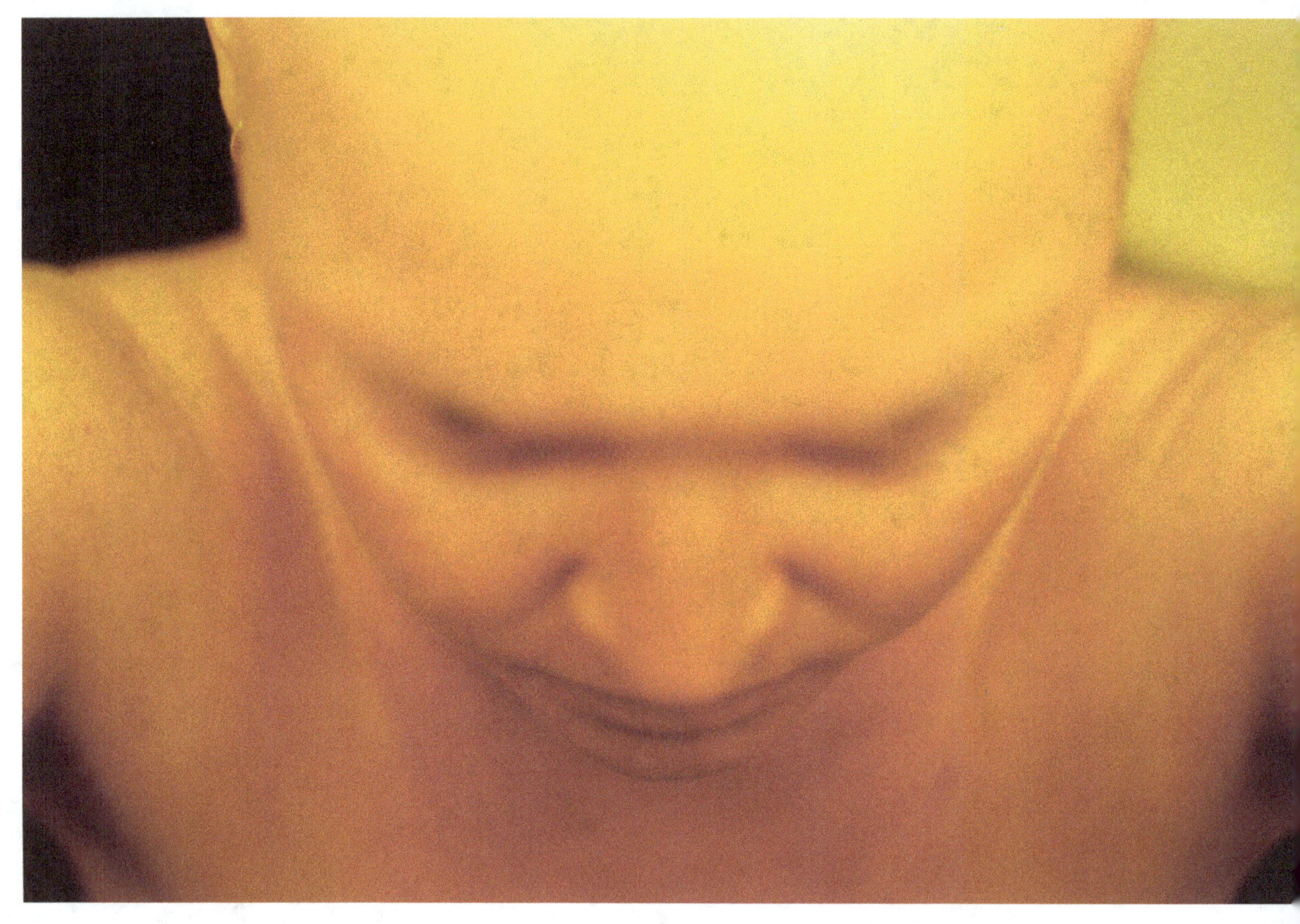

16

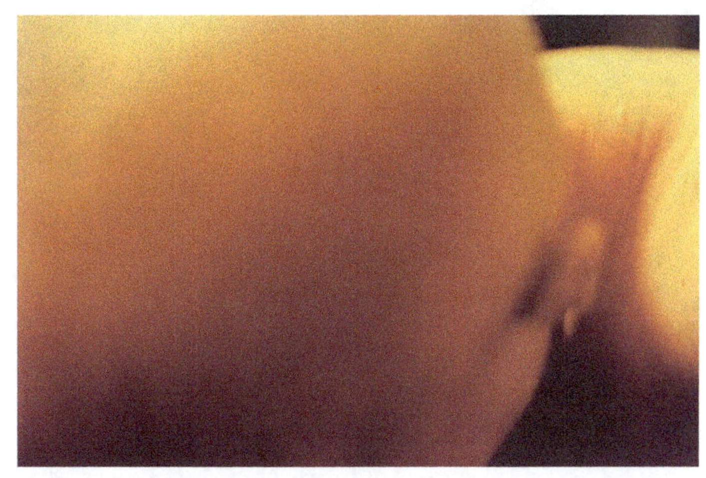

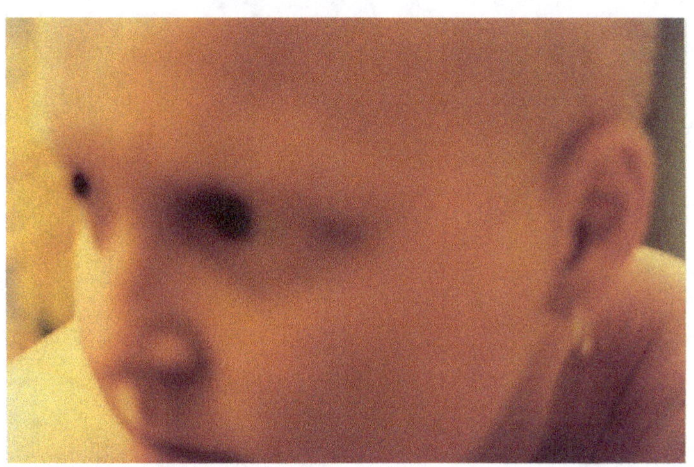

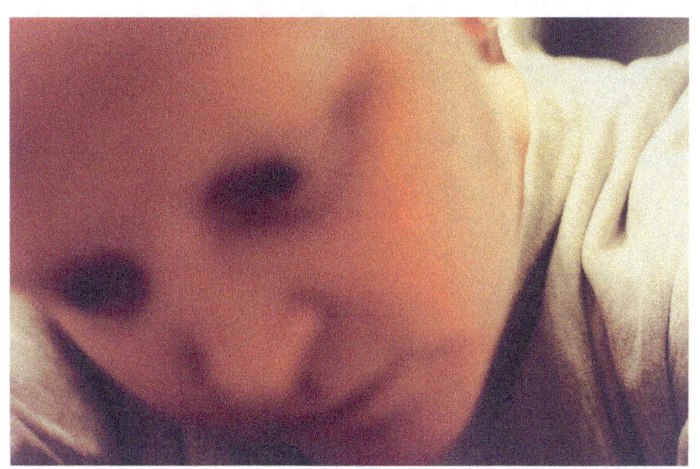

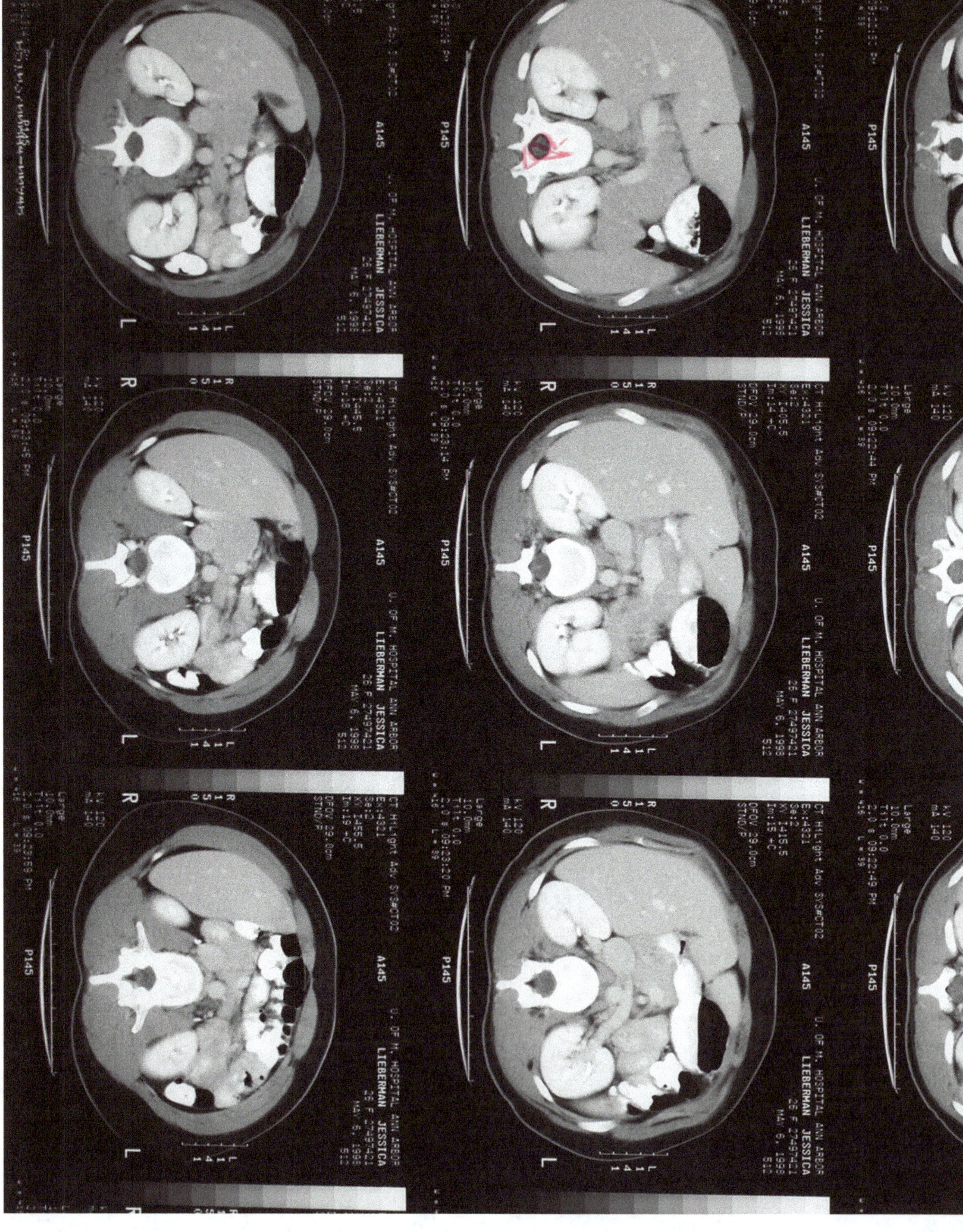

ONSET

It was in my groin, on the left side, and felt like a pulled muscle or some other kind of reaction to the ridiculous poses I inanely struck in yoga class. Yoga was a vague attempt at insisting upon the continuing presence of my physical body, despite all evidence to the contrary. Eating and sleeping were performed when convenient and had little correspondence with any kind of biological desire or need. Pain too—headaches, backaches, heartaches—went unnoticed. The dissertation was to be the new body, the body of my own creation, and my sack of flesh and bones and hair was to be sacrificed in its honor, a willing penitent to a loftier purpose. And so the pain that woke me at 3:14 on that March morning should have been an infuriating nuisance, a nagging detail that prevented me from using my time wisely and recuperating my strength for a few precious hours so that I might return, clearheaded, to my words. But somehow it was not. The pain did not work its way into the haze, joining yoga and roughage as they labored unnoticed to remind me that my life expanded beyond the corpus of my writing task. Instead, this pain snapped me awake suddenly and held me at attention until months later, when I finally convinced a doctor that something was wrong. And then, as if vanquished, the awareness, the clarity, passed. I had done my job somehow. Gotten the attention of the experts who would now make all decisions about my physical needs and activities for me. My body's fate was scripted now, fitting into a regimented system of doctor's visits,

blood draws, CT scans, chemotherapy treatments, radiation
treatments, and handling of side effects. So, as if it knew
its services were no longer required, my focus vanished
and left me to a new kind of haze—the murky newness of
myself as yet unwritten: myself as cancer patient.

And now these two bodies of mine—the long-haired and
exercised body that I had put on hold, and the body of my
book—a body that I labored tediously to mold and form—
are memories. Both will return, I know that. But even when
they do, even when I am "cured," each body can never
again be taken for granted. I will always know that both of
these bodies (once so clearly separate, mingling only in my
most repressed musings) were lost and regained: lost for-
ever in their inevitability and to be regained only as possibilities. These bodies are not of this present time. They are
of the past and the future. For now, my body is something
else . . . something I cannot even begin to imagine.

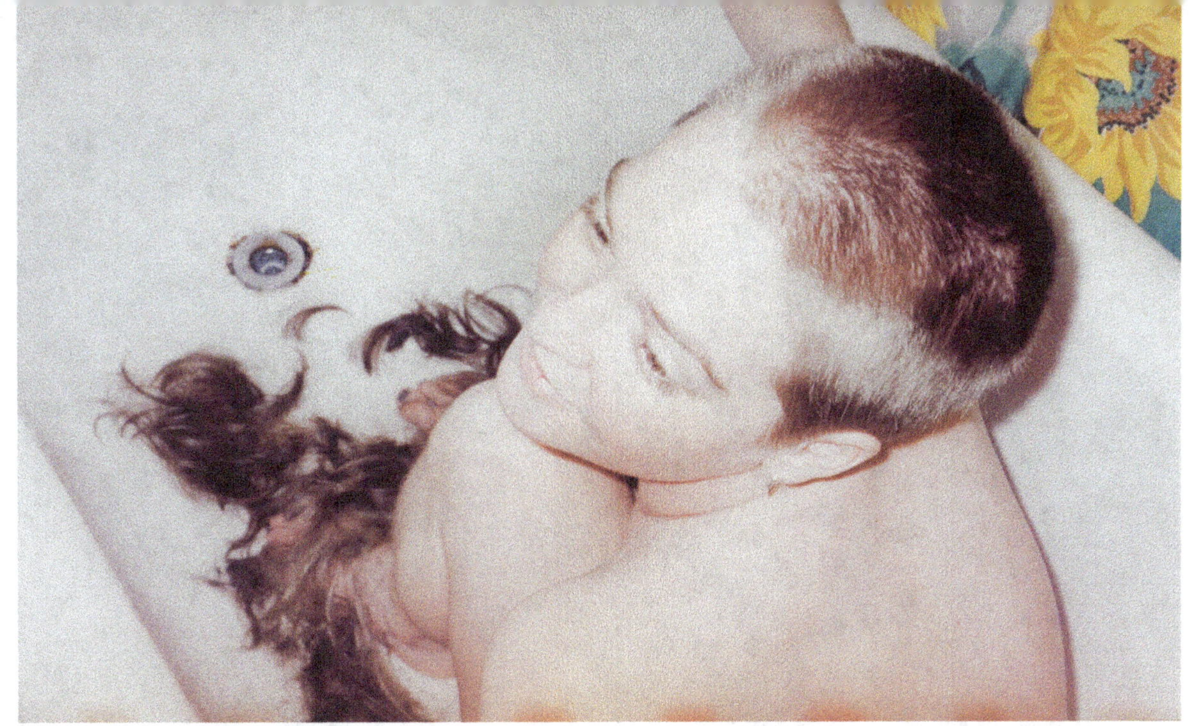

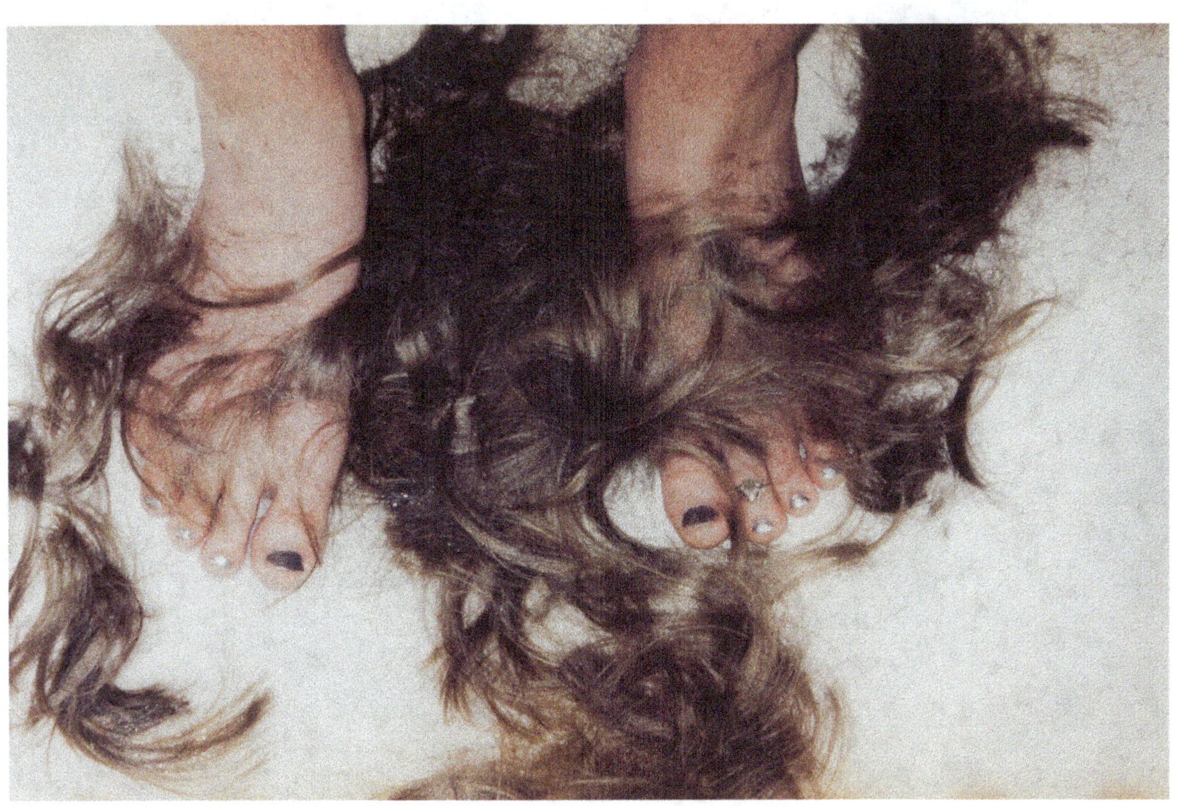

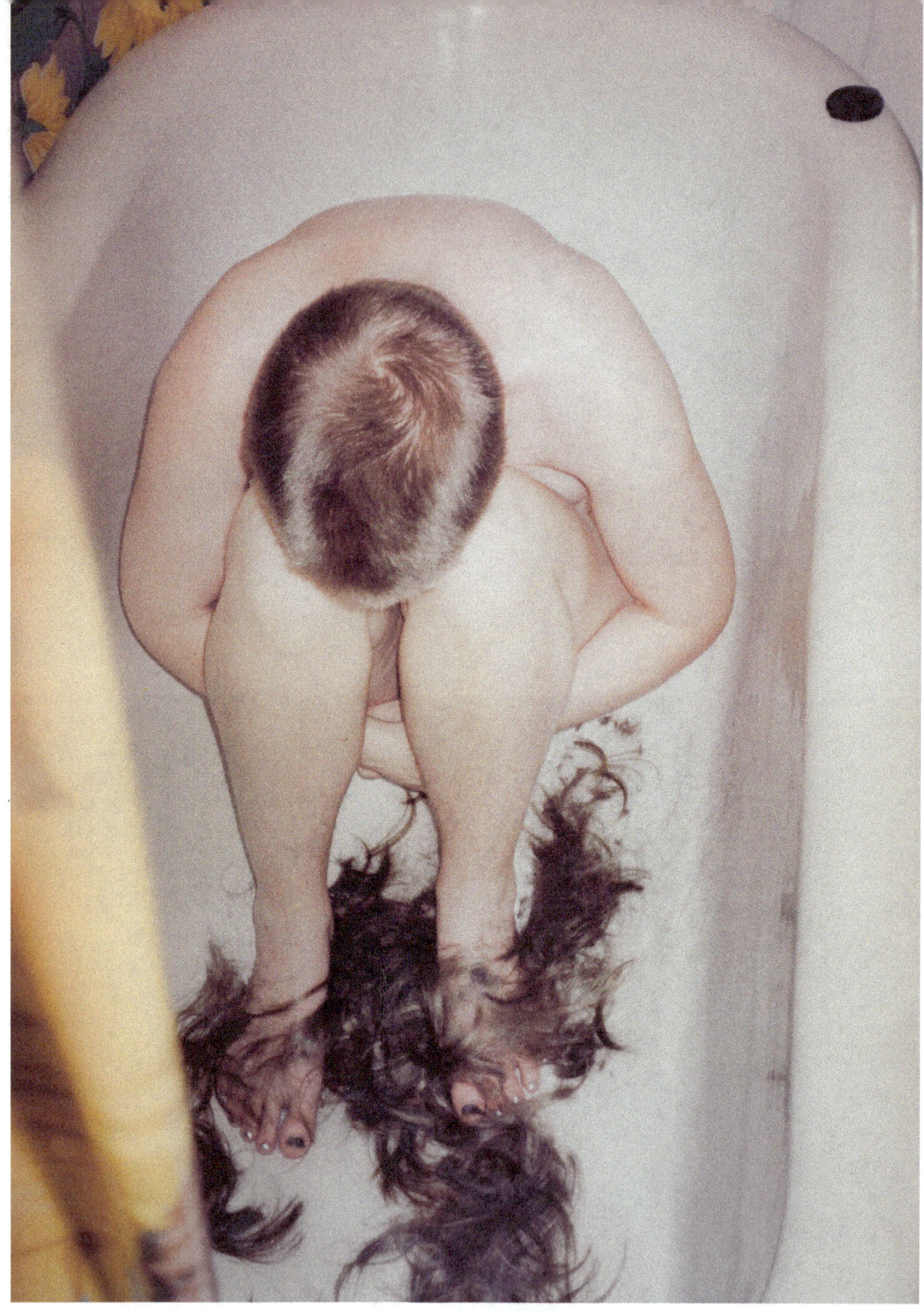

24

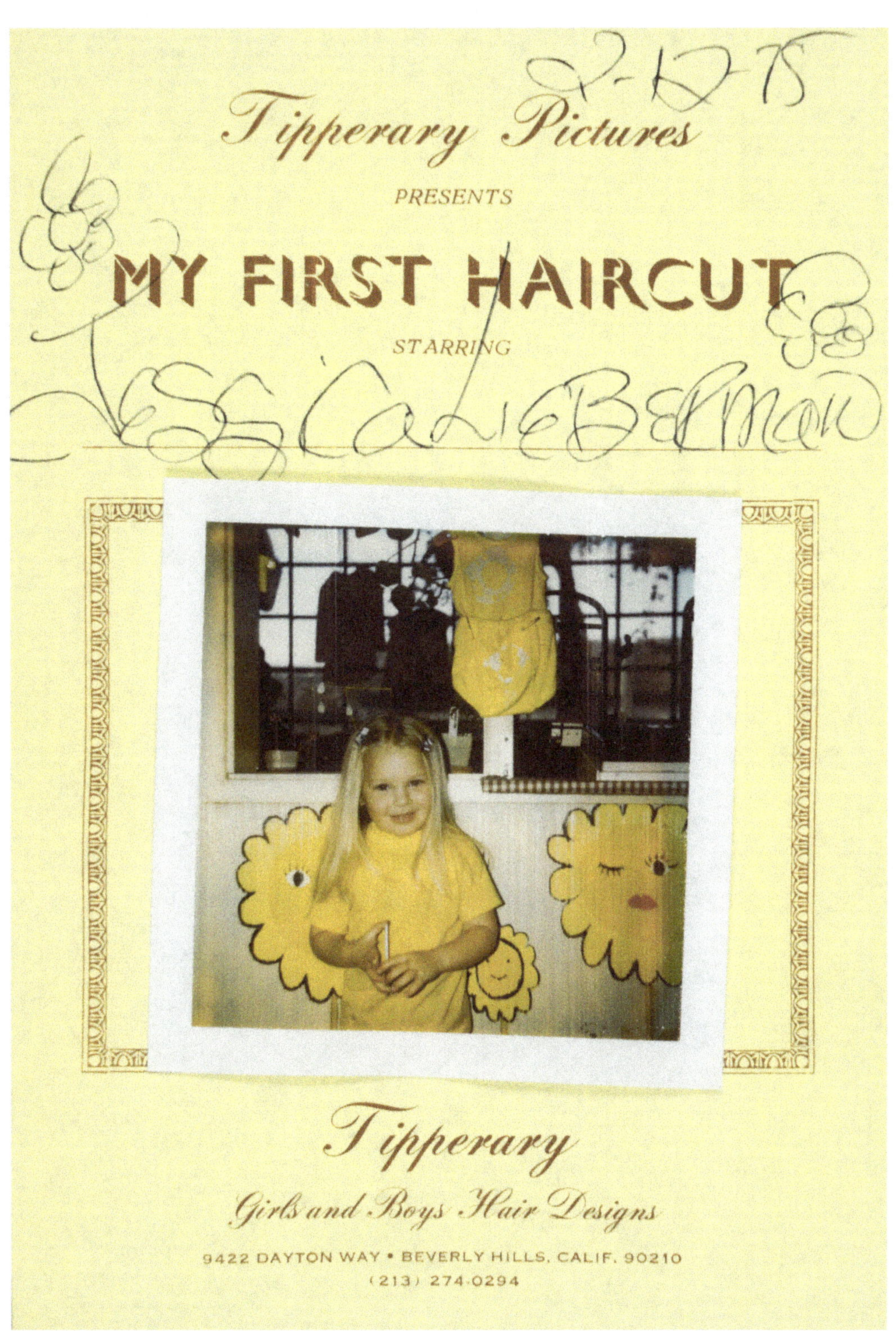
2-12-75
Tipperary Pictures
PRESENTS
MY FIRST HAIRCUT
STARRING
JESSICA LIEBERMAN
Tipperary
Girls and Boys Hair Designs
9422 DAYTON WAY • BEVERLY HILLS, CALIF. 90210
(213) 274-0294

Words

In 1998 I was diagnosed with Cancer.

Seems a simple statement, and yet not a bit of that sentence, once written, rings true. Not because I cannot recognize the truth of my physical situation. On the contrary, awareness-recognition-acceptance is an unavoidable process when your body fails you. There is no option for denial when you are puking up the only ounces of food you have managed to swallow in days—food you fought hard to get past your shredded esophagus—food that burned and stung going down even though your brain acknowledges that it is smooth, soothing applesauce. Staring at it now, in the toilet bowl, that rejected applesauce appears almost a blessing—at least you won't find yourself in a bone-marrow transplant bed, with a sleepily distant nurse forcing enema mixture into your bloated and agonizing insides—all in a desperate attempt to pass that damned sustenance. In such a state, believe me, you know you are sick—know exactly what you have, how it is pronounced, how it is treated, how it used to be treated, how it may be treated in the future. You know its scientific name, its diagnostic criteria, its differential diagnosis, its cellular structure, its statistical success at killing people.

The problem with that simple sentence is its simplicity; its certainty; its clarity. There is nothing in its linguistic container that at all represents my experience of illness.

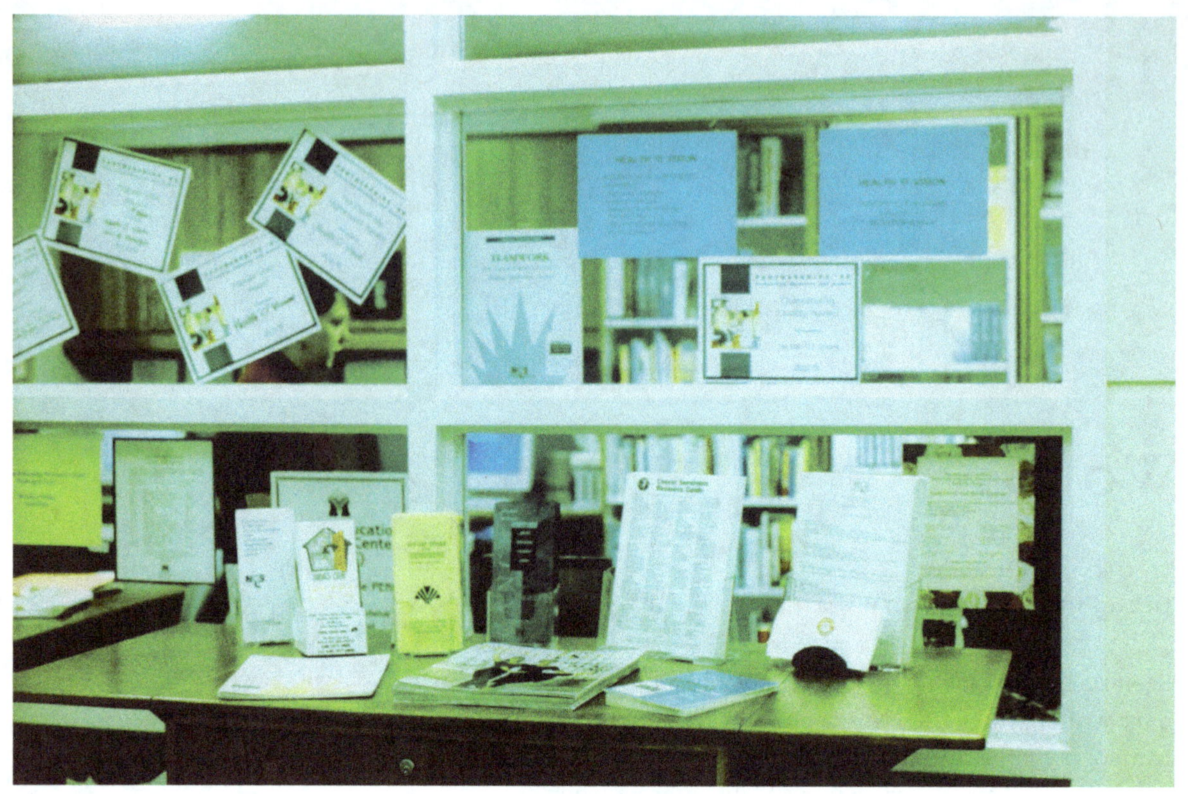

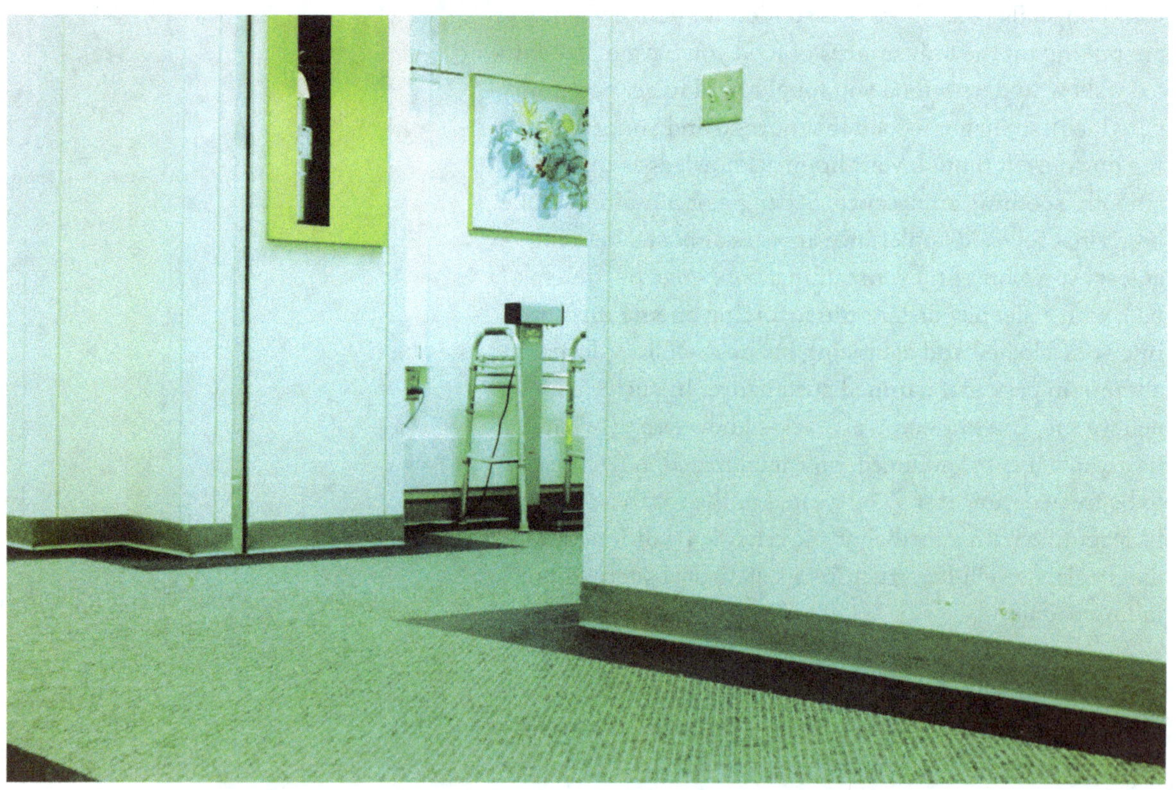

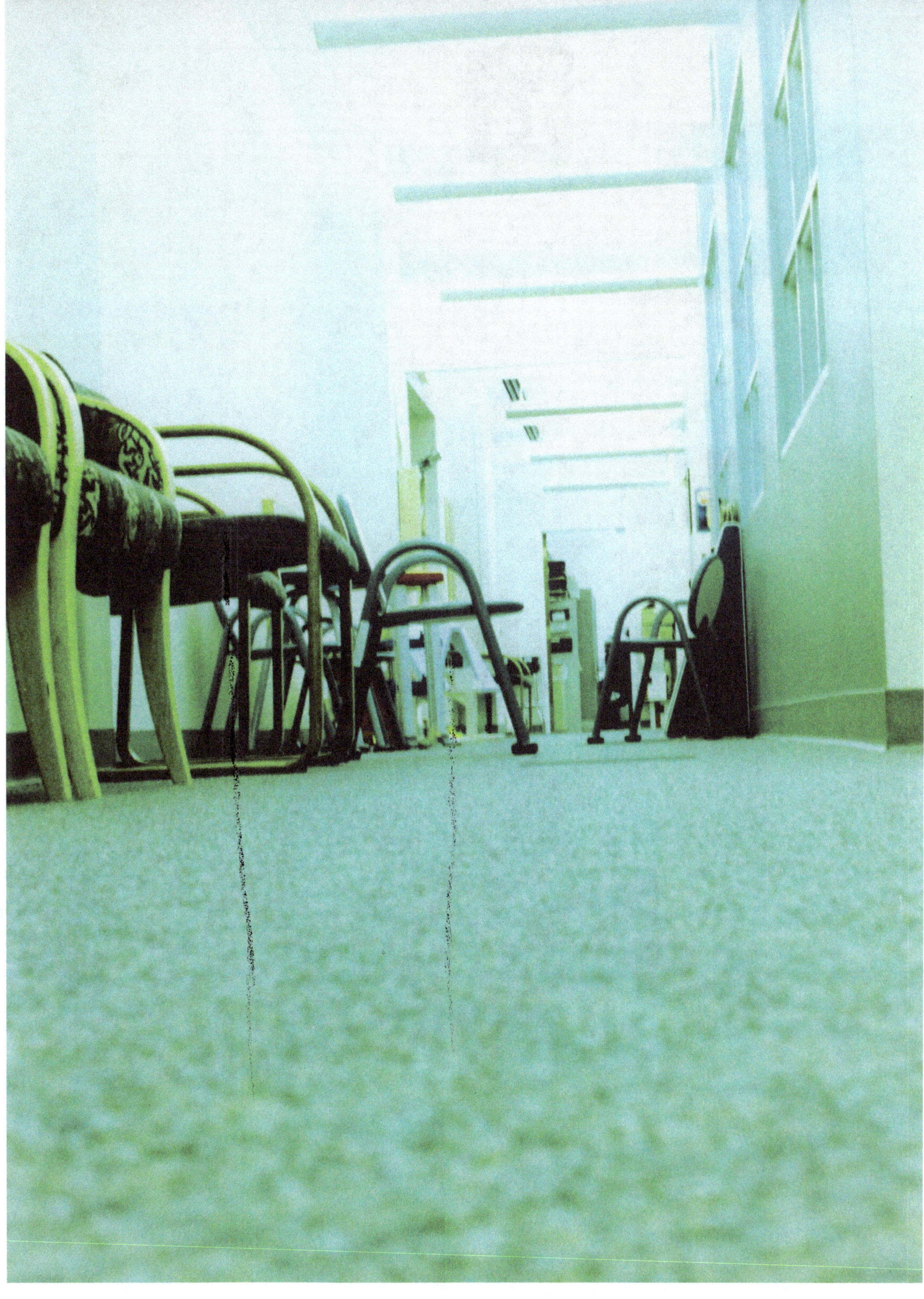

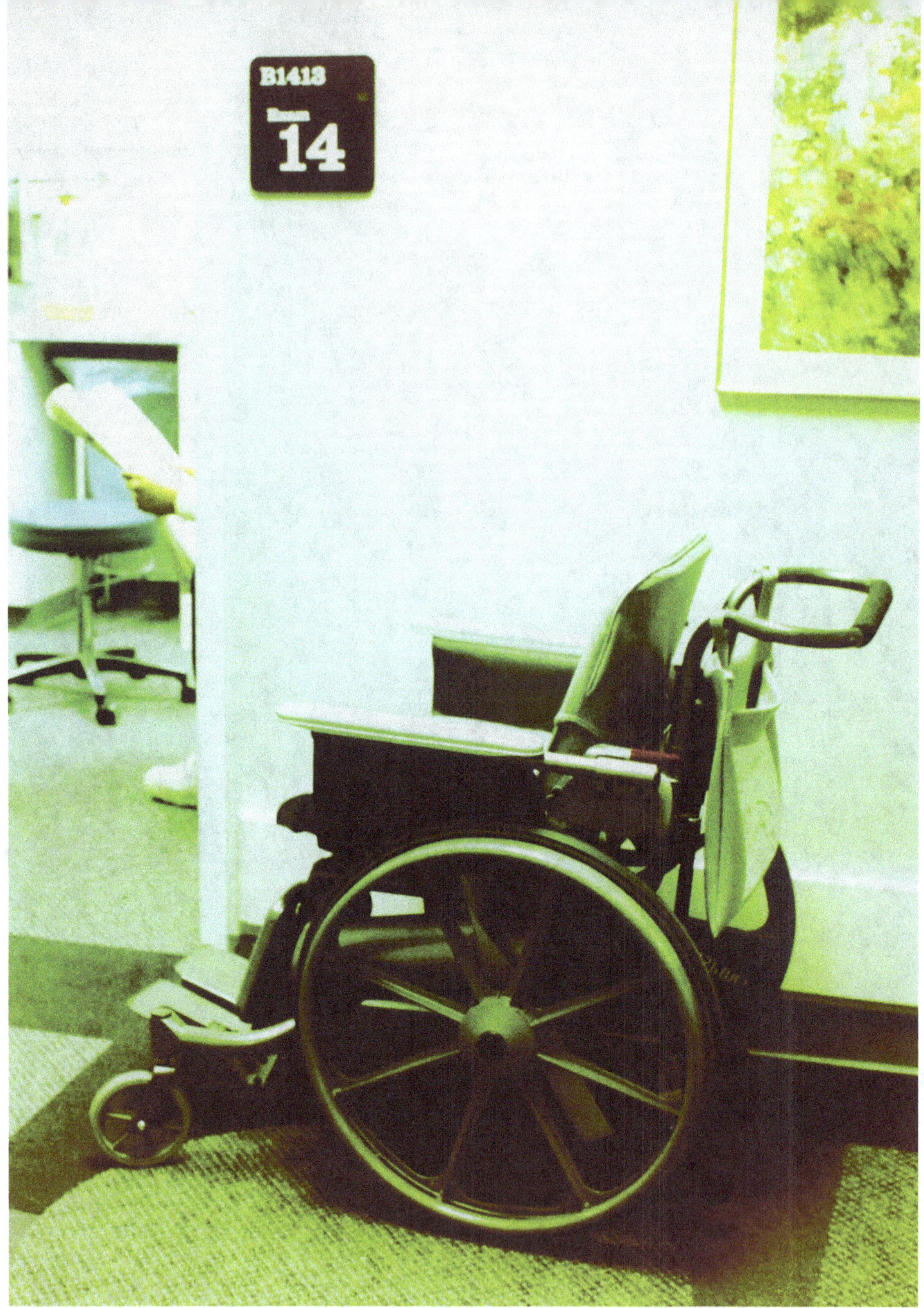

B1413
Room
14

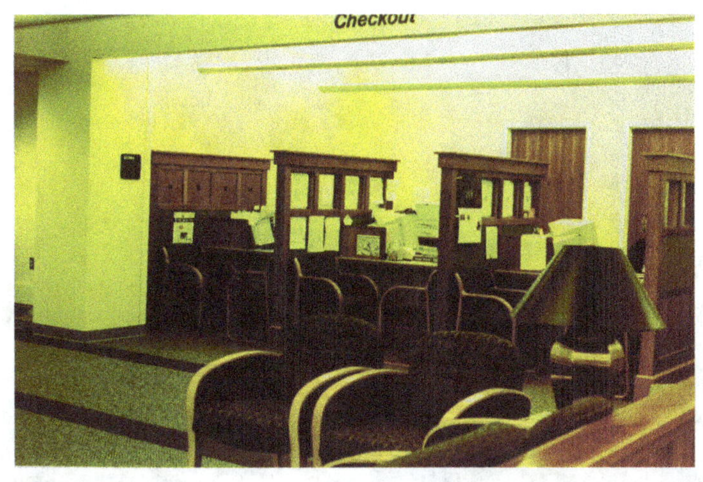

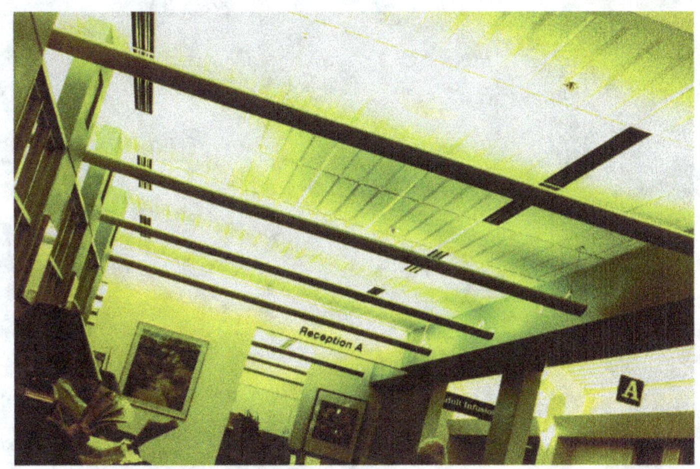

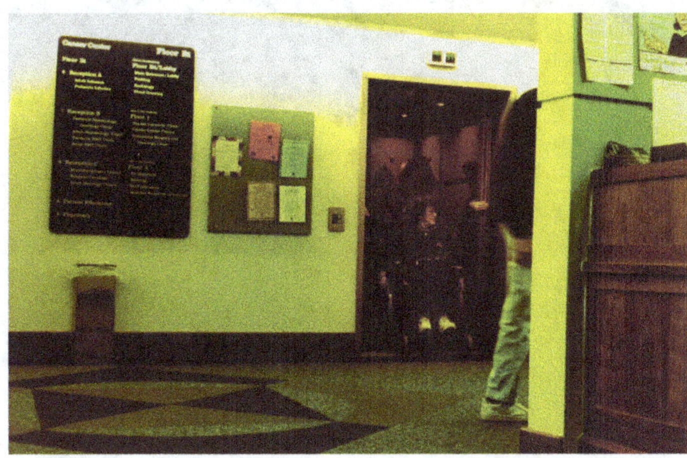

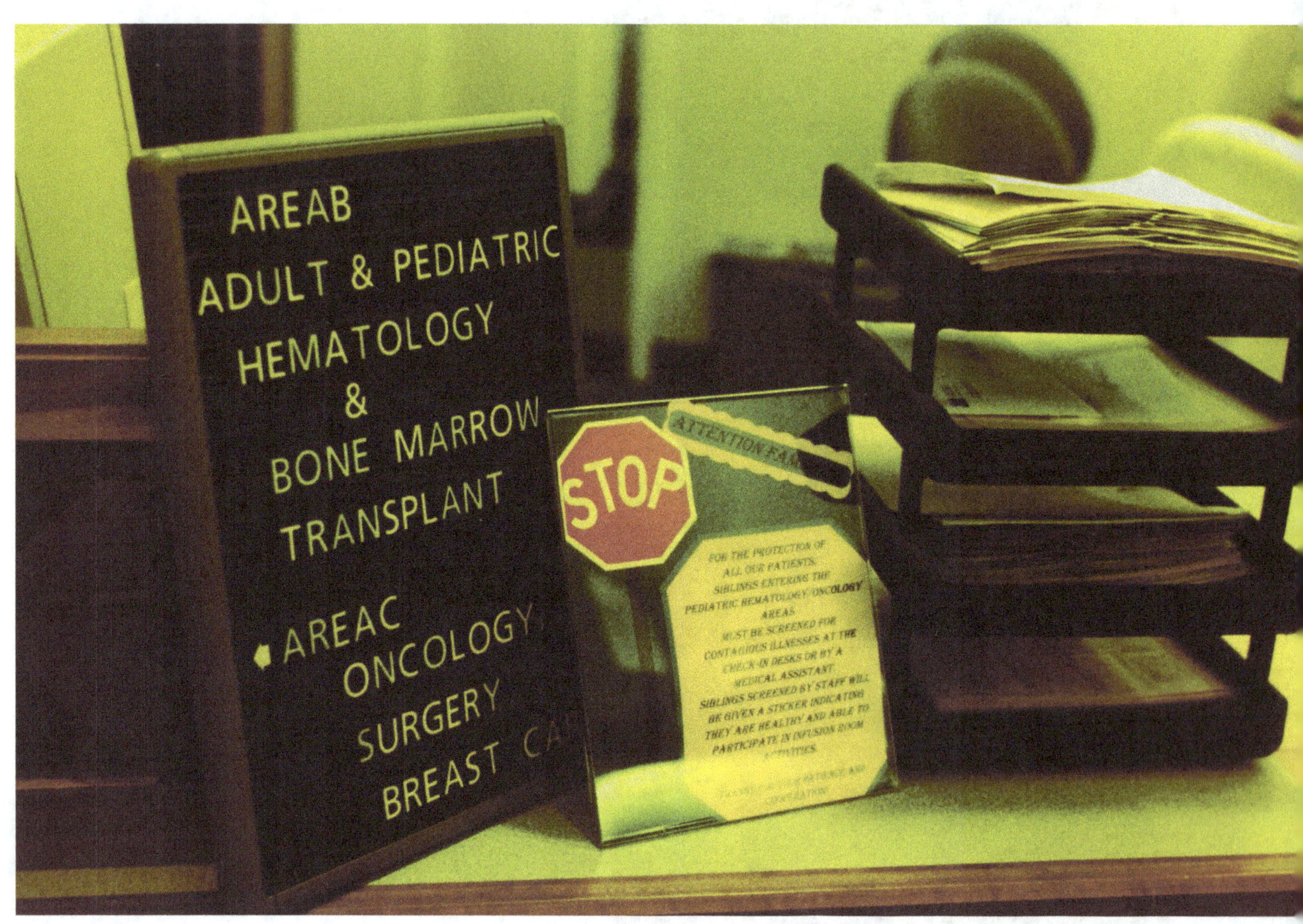
AREAB
ADULT & PEDIATRIC
HEMATOLOGY
&
BONE MARROW
TRANSPLANT

AREAC
ONCOLOGY
SURGERY
BREAST CA

STOP
ATTENTION FAM

FOR THE PROTECTION OF
ALL OUR PATIENTS,
SIBLINGS ENTERING THE
PEDIATRIC HEMATOLOGY/ONCOLOGY
AREAS
MUST BE SCREENED FOR
CONTAGIOUS ILLNESSES AT THE
CHECK-IN DESKS OR BY A
MEDICAL ASSISTANT.
SIBLINGS SCREENED BY STAFF WILL
BE GIVEN A STICKER INDICATING
THEY ARE HEALTHY AND ABLE TO
PARTICIPATE IN INFUSION ROOM
ACTIVITIES.

Support

LAST WEEK A FRIEND ASKED ME FOR A PROFOUND REVELATION, a great lesson that I was learning from my Cancer Experience. He wanted to hear that it had changed my life, re-ordered my priorities, made me recognize the truth I had been missing. I had nothing to give him.

Changing his approach, he then asked if I had joined any support groups. I laughed. I had no interest in them. I believed in their value—but only for other people. I had my own community of support. As for a community of sick people, these groups seemed artificial, forced, composed out of desperation.

But when I passed the Cancer Center's "information library" at my next appointment, I looked at the list of support groups anyway. There were three for caretakers, one for the elderly, one for children, two for adolescents, and nine for breast cancer patients or survivors. None for me.

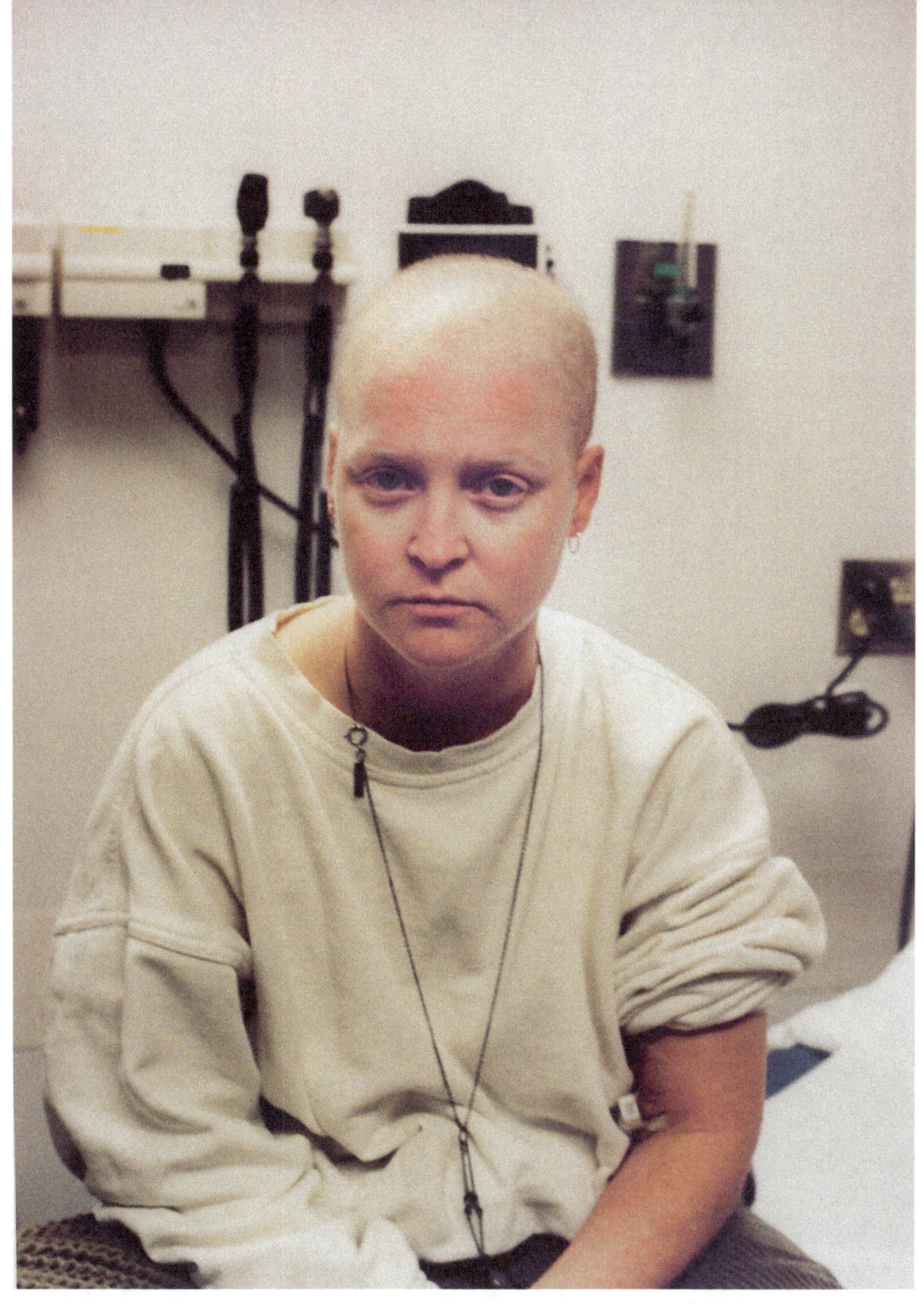

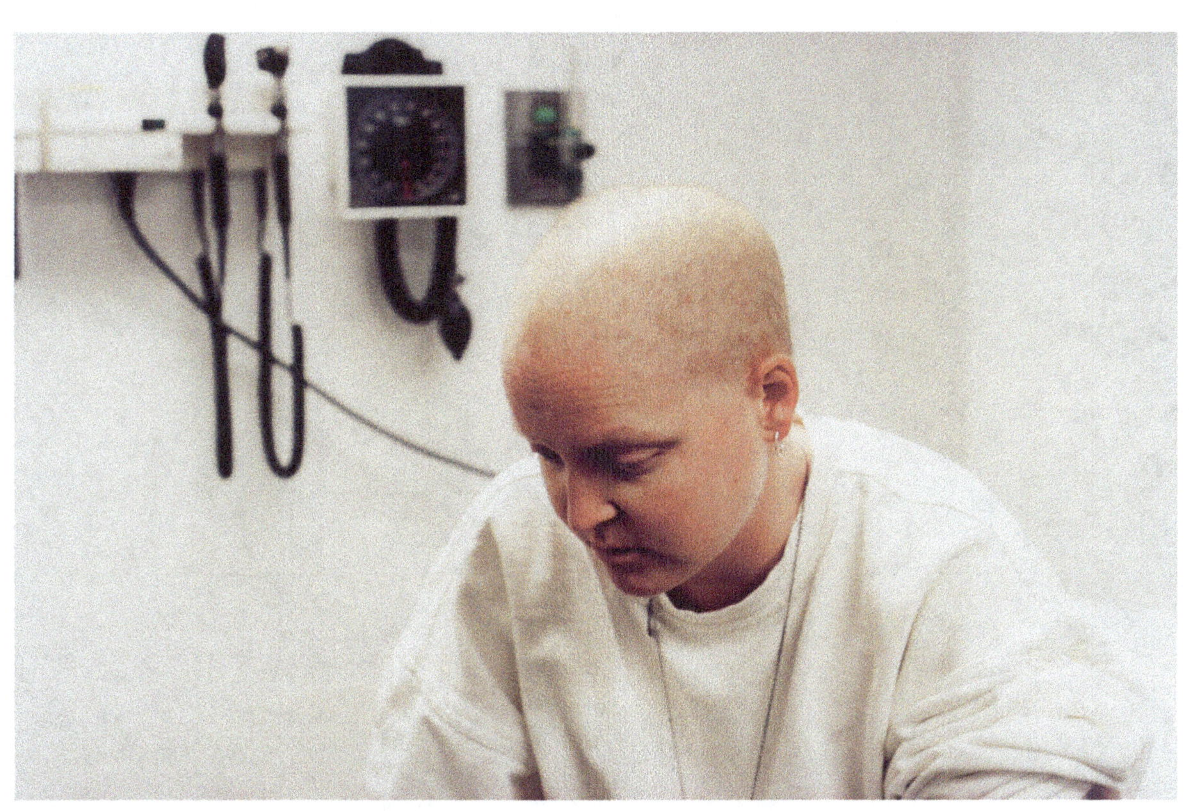

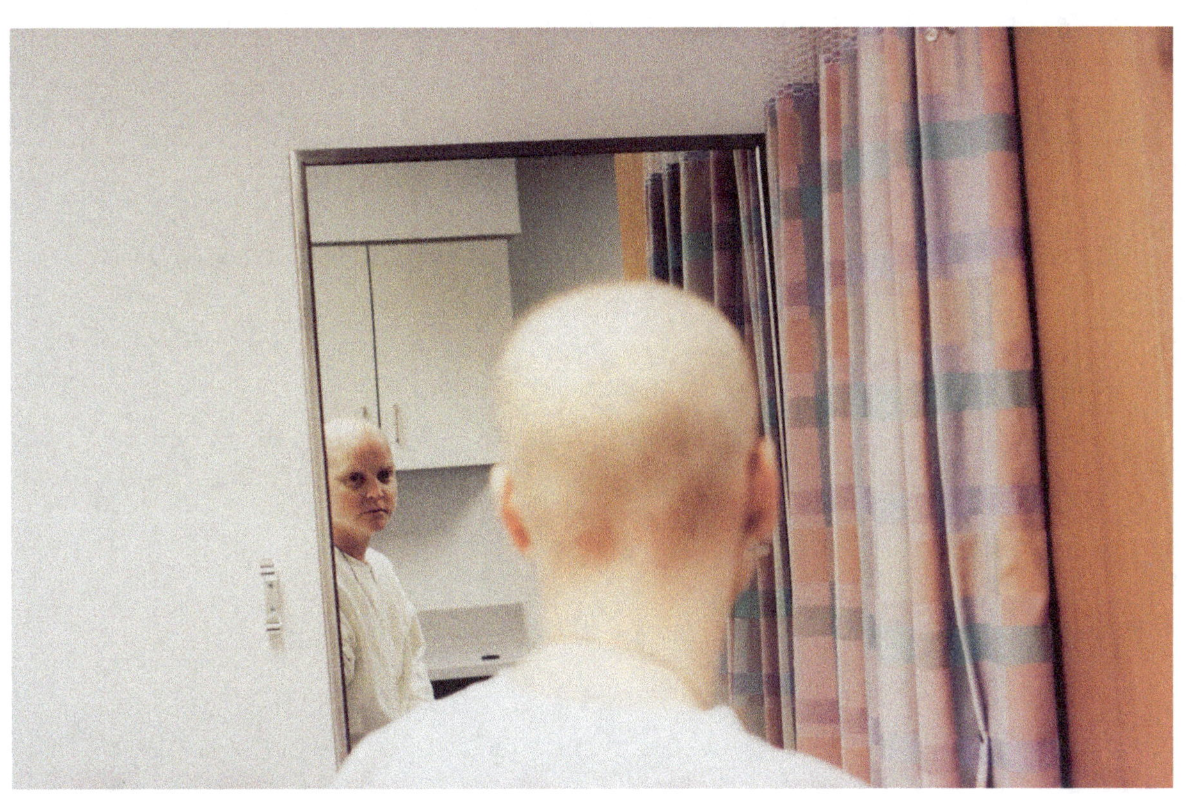

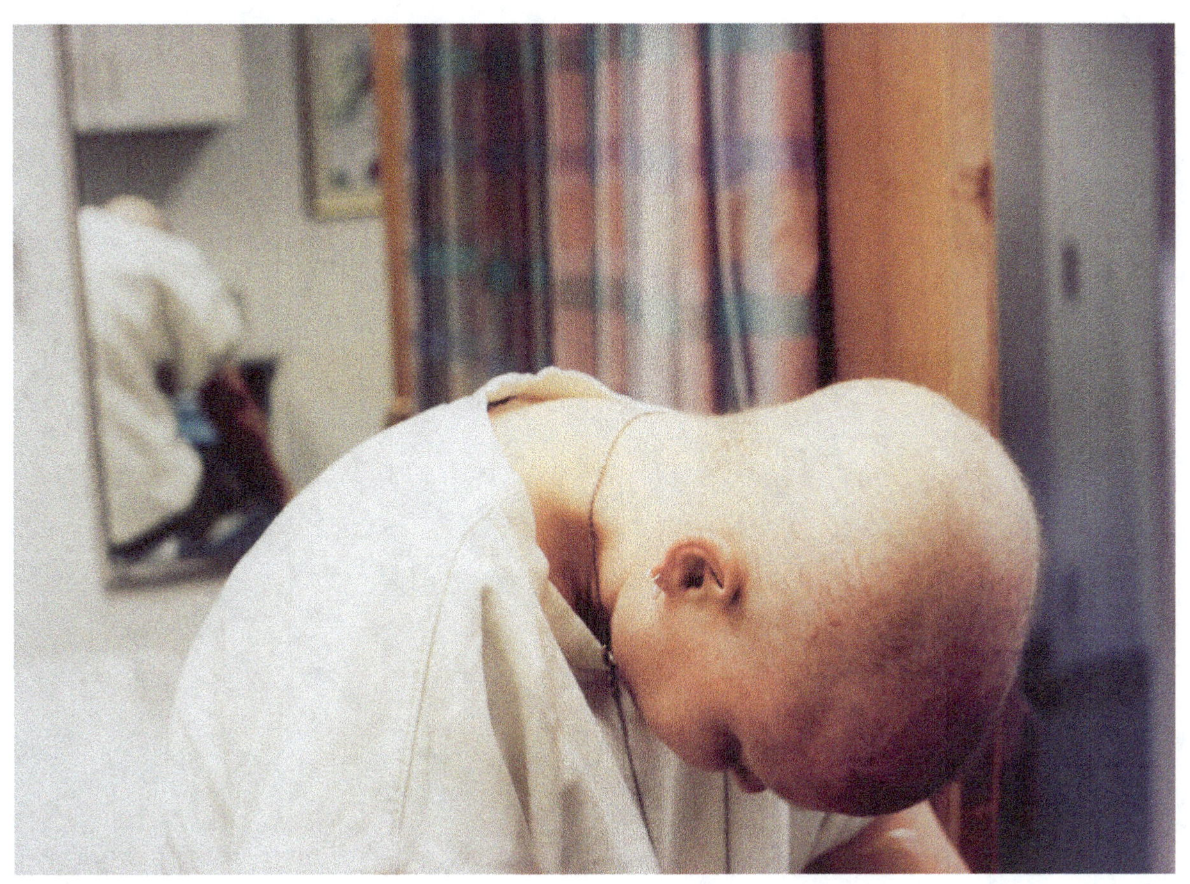

Invisible

I wonder if they have any idea what waiting around in waiting rooms and examination rooms means to a sick person.

I wait a half hour to have my blood drawn, two to three hours to see my doctor, and an hour for my chemotherapy treatment to be prepared. All together, my regular visit takes about six to seven hours—at least half of the time is spent in the waiting room.

Waiting for my doctor today, I struck up a conversation with a man in the examination room across from mine. We were both sitting there alone, silently, impatiently waiting. After several minutes of glancing at one another, making eye contact, smiling and looking away, I finally commented on his hair. It was clearly growing back, a sure sign of his having recently finished his chemo regimen. He beamed at me and unleashed a mini-torrent of exclamations: No one had ever broken the awkward "waiting room silence" with him before; he had always wanted to talk with his fellow "waiters" but had never dared; he was ashamed of his curiosity; he feared their bitterness; he feared his own; what did I have? "Oh really! Me too! But I'm in remission now and all the . . ."

He was cut off—my doctor arrived, told us we shouldn't be talking with one another, and shut both our doors.

TREATMENT

I only called my mom from "the chair" because I knew
that this was really good news, news I was supposed to be
excited and relieved by, news I was supposed to share.
I called a friend immediately after, reasoning that I might
as well use my cell phone's prepaid monthly minutes, but
knowing really that I would not be able to think about this
new x-ray much longer. If I were going to get the news
out, it would have to be right then, while I was enveloped
in the chair, still focused on the biweekly responsibility of
my appointment and its paraphernalia. Once I got home
I would sleep till Saturday and would awake needing to
feel like Jessica, my duties to Cancer Jessica having been
accomplished for the time being. But by Sunday I would
be sick again, bombarded with banal side effects for sure,
perhaps facing any number of more serious discomforts
that always seemed to land me in urgent care. And this fact
does not seem to trouble anyone but me: I can only just
bear to mention such minor maladies to my partner, feeling wholly incapable of actually calling my doctor. Calling
my hematologist to alert him to my sore throat, I find
myself fighting the urge to announce to him that I have
also found a small but noisy fly in my apartment. This is
why this week's good news provides me with not an ounce
of relief or enthusiasm. Really I don't feel anything about
it at all, except a little annoyance at having to sound excited
when relaying the information. Otherwise, thinking about
it now, I guess I just feel a little numb.

OK, and perhaps I am somewhat exasperated by the
expectation that I should be so relieved. Why? Because
one of my tumors is shrinking, disappearing off of the
computer screen in a doctor's office? Because the treatment is "working"? If every single person's response to my
cancer was to add another line to a rousing chorus of "Oh
that's OK, not a problem, my friend had that and he/she
is totally fine, I'll give you his/her number," then what's
the surprise? The few friends who didn't have a verse to
add to the song of assurance quickly called back to revise
their previous fear and sorrow with alleviating statistics
freshly downloaded from the Internet. Filing away a bar-
rage of letters and photocopies announcing expectations
for my cure rate, I felt too tired to answer the phone as the
machine ventriloquized yet another friendly but unknown
voice offering to share their saga of illness and inevitable
health, sagas that so affected our mutual acquaintance
and thus required our introduction. Relief to me is when
the answering machine relays a familiar voice calling
to tell of their own good news. Relief to me is when the
twelve messages don't all turn out to be from the blood
lab. I am relieved to speak to friends who are interested in
my teaching or my research, relieved to talk with lifetime
buddies who are overwhelmed with their own life plans.
Lou's engagement, Jon's wedding, Tina's baby, Molly's
troublesome boyfriend, Kellie's three children, Jordan's
shitty job: now those are a relief. Whether the tumors
are dying or not, it's still July and the earache and metal
mouth that woke me up this morning aren't going anywhere until December at the earliest. It sounds crass, but
the only new news the images on the computer screen
provided was that the Cancer Center's radiology department now scanned x-rays directly onto disc, whereas I had
wandered the freezing halls of the hospital's basement to
pick up x-rays that scanned into the computer as a giant
blob of white on a gray background. Of course, this news
didn't help my artistic endeavors anyway—I was informed
that I was not allowed to have a copy of these beautifully
scanned images of my insides.

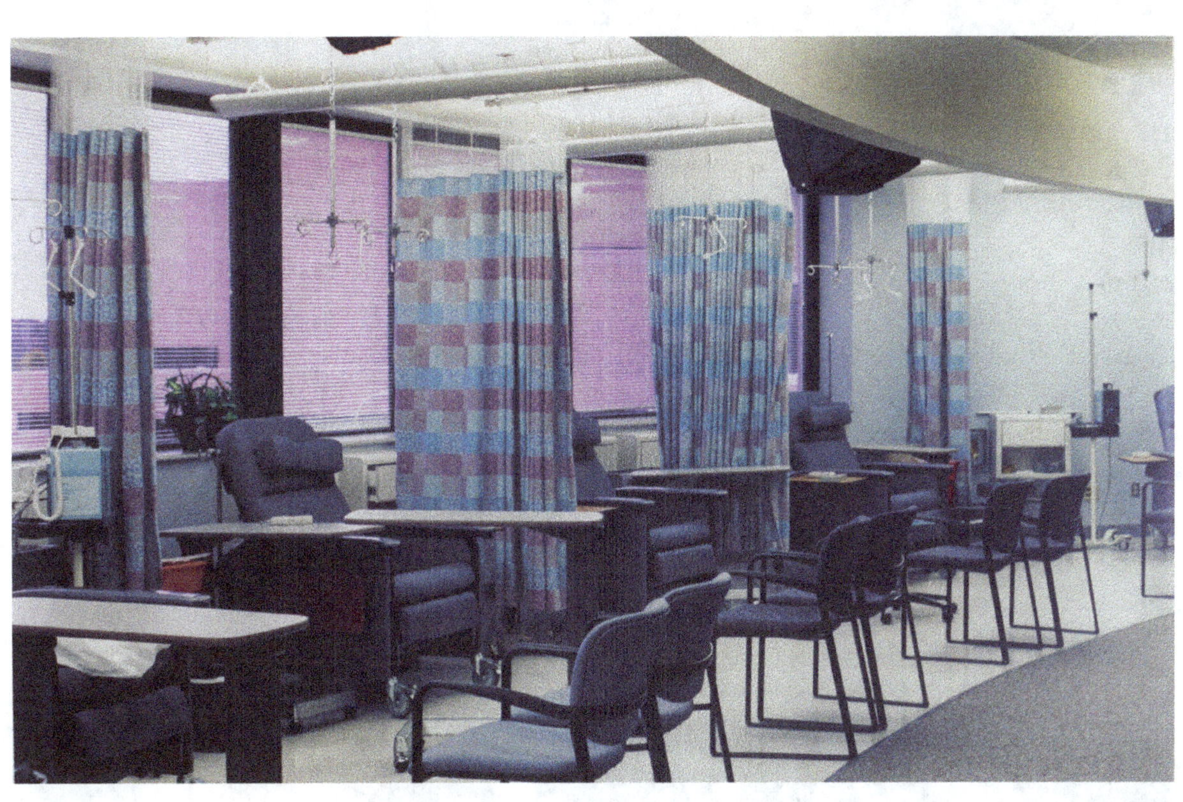

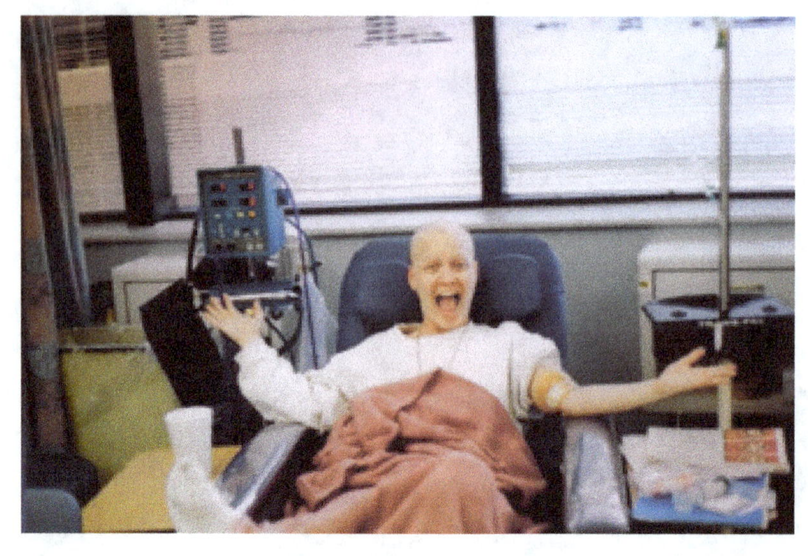

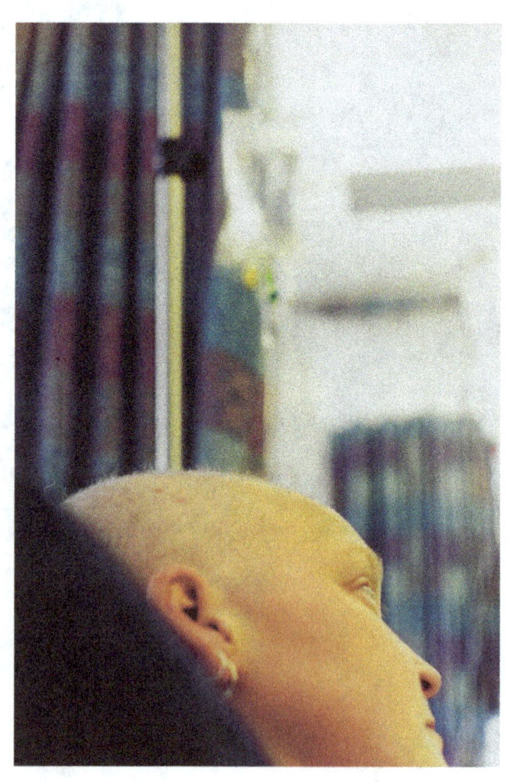

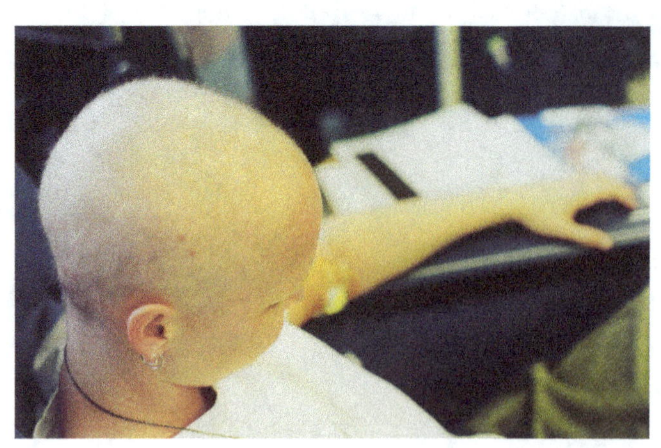

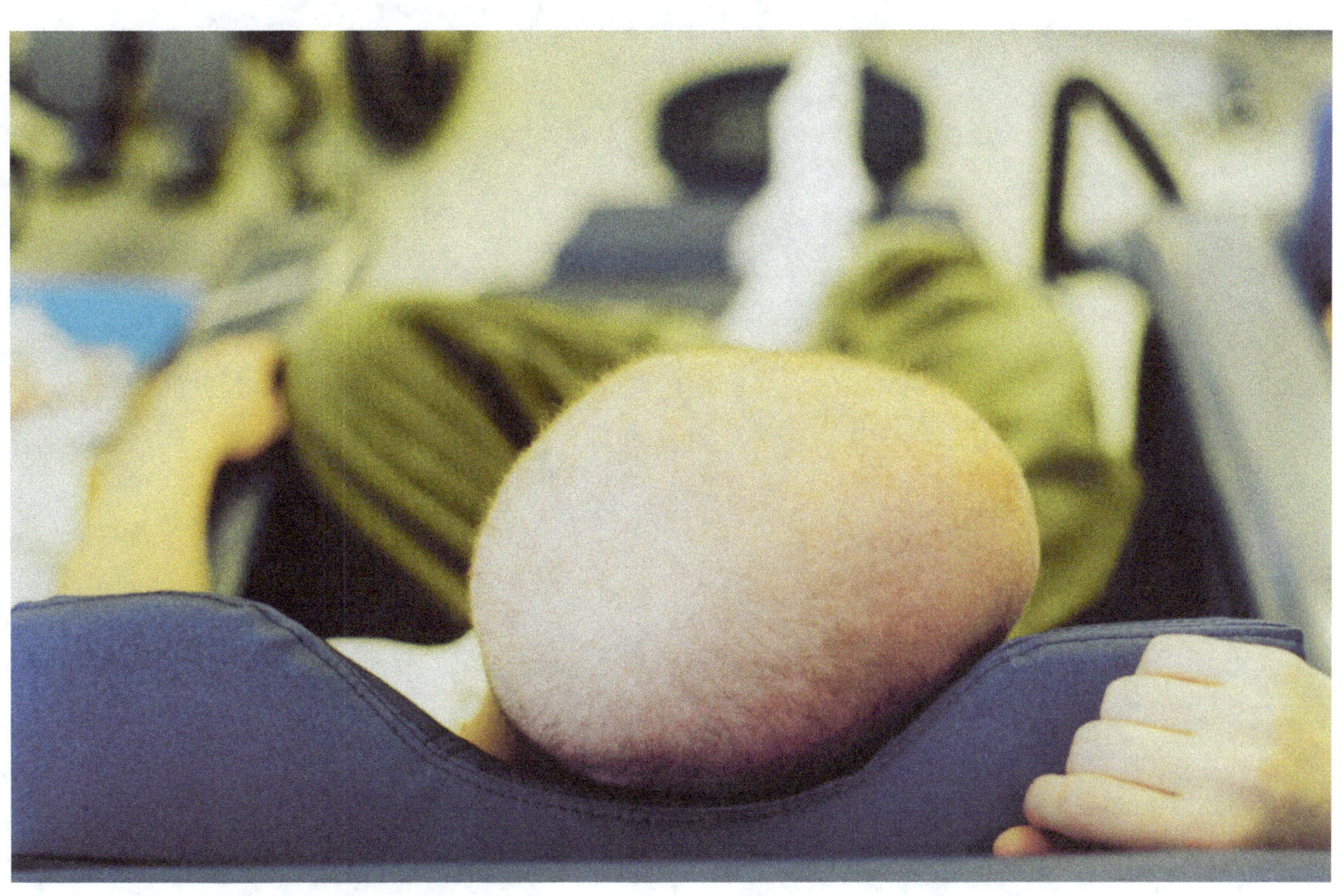

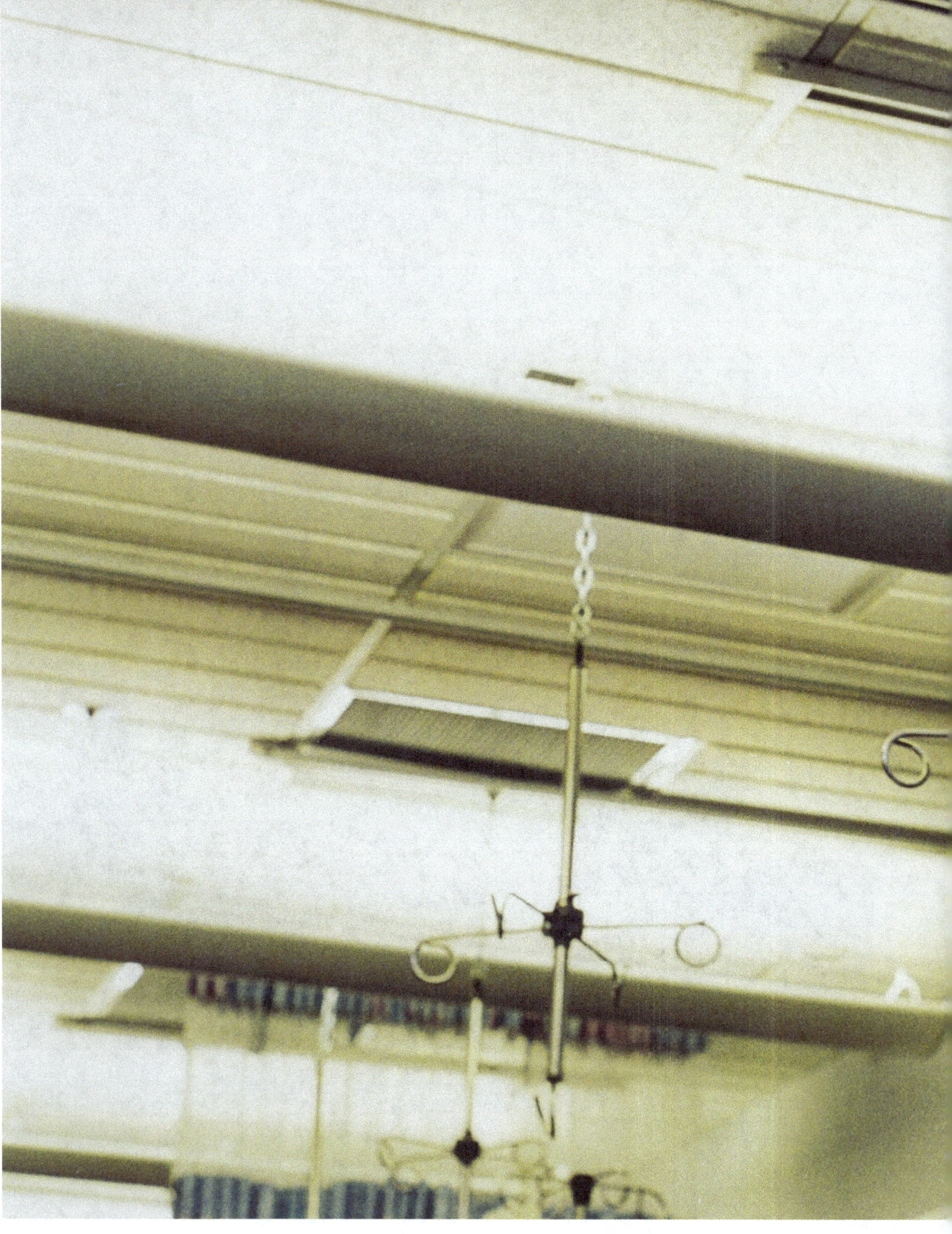

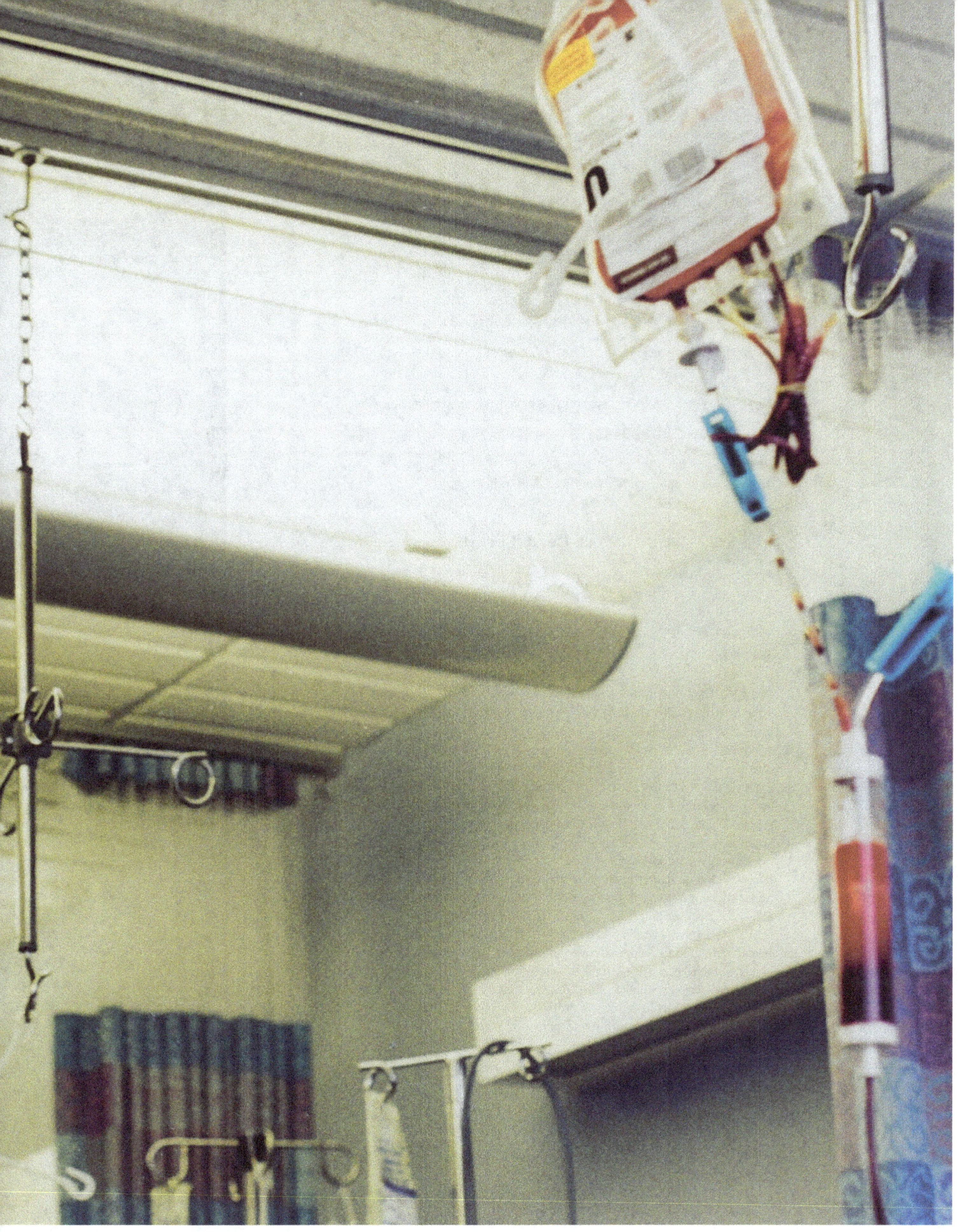

It was a pleasure to see your patient today in the Medical Procedures Unit for a fiberoptic bronchoscopy, transbronchial lung biopsy, and Wang needle aspirate of the lung.

Indications: The patient has mediastinal adenopathy, multiple arthralgias, and a question of sarcoidosis.

The patient was prepared in the usual manner with 4% lidocaine used to inject the vocal cords and 2% below. She received 100 mg of fentanyl for conscious sedation and 3 mg of Versed.

The right lower lobe was transbronchially biopsied times 5, and good pieces were obtained. At the main carina, because of the mediastinal silhouette, the patient did have a Wang needle aspirate times two. Slides were smeared with cell fixatives and sent to the Pathology Lab.

Lavaged fluid was sent for appropriate cytology and microbiology studies.

The patient tolerated the procedure extremely well. A chest x-ray was obtained and is pending at the time of this dictation.

Thanks again for allowing us to participate in the patient's care.

PREOPERATIVE DIAGNOSIS: Cervical lymphadenopathy, possible lymphoma.

POSTOPERATIVE DIAGNOSIS: Same.

OPERATION PERFORMED: Excision of cervical lymph nodes of the right neck.

PROCEDURE: With the patient supine in the Operating Room and the head turned towards the left, the right neck was prepped and draped so that a supraclavicular incision could be made over the two heads of the sternocleidomastoid muscle. The incision was about 3 1/2 cm. long and carried through the skin, subcutaneum and the platysma muscle. Hemostasis was obtained and an incision was made in the fascia between the two heads of the sternocleidomastoid muscle allowing dissection into the supraclavicular deeper space, after which two enlarged lymph nodes were readily palpable and with sharp and blunt dissection these were freed from surrounding tissue. The largest of the nodes was about 3 cm. in diameter and the smaller of the two was about 2 x 2 cm. in diameter. These were removed without difficulty, and hemostasis was obtained. Several stitches of 4-0 Vicryl were used to reapproximate the fascia between the muscle heads and the same was used for the platysma muscle layer and these were buried. Stitches of 4-0 silk were used to approximate the skin, after which a dry sterile dressing was applied, and the patient was allowed to return home ambulating freely.

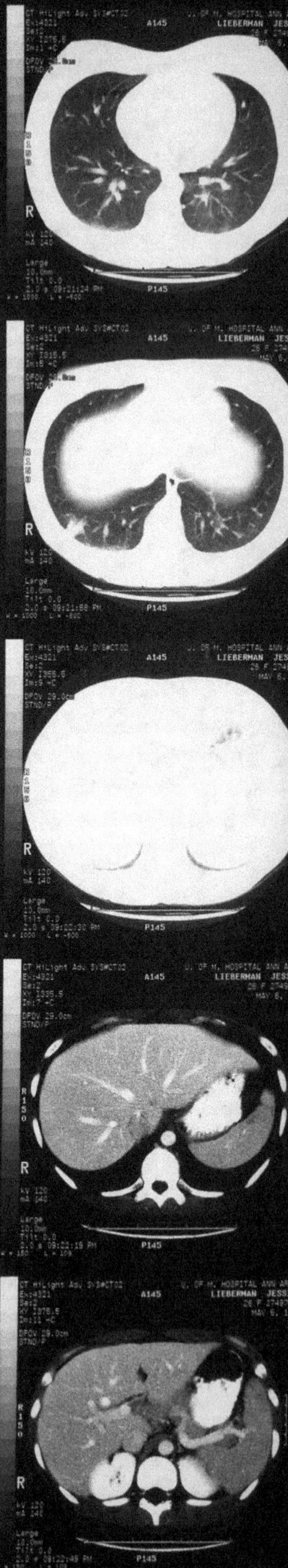

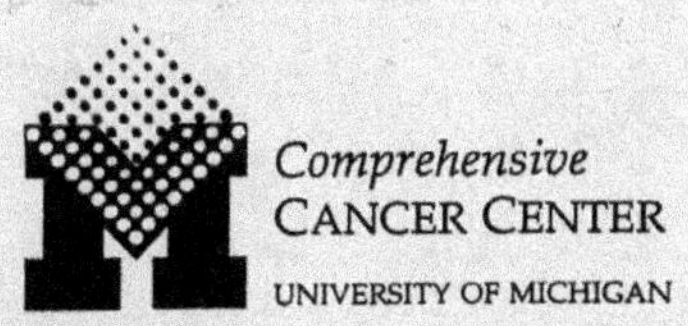

Robert Winfield, M.D.
207 Fletcher
Ann Arbor, MI 48105

Dear Dr. Winfield:

We had the pleasure of meeting Ms. Jessica Lieberman in our Hematology Clinic today, May 29, 1998. As you are aware, she is a 26-year-old female who was recently diagnosed with Hodgkin's disease. Her symptoms began in March of 1998 at which time she developed arthralgias, fevers to approximately 101 degrees, and drenching night sweats. These were treated with Aleve and Indocin with mild resolution. She also has developed substantial itching to the point where she is excoriating her skin. She also reports development of photosensitivity at this time, rash, aphthous ulcers, and Raynaud's phenomena of her upper extremities and ears. She was seen by the Rheumatology Department here at the University of Michigan Medical Center by Dr. Kazmers. Prior evaluation included a chest x-ray which demonstrated a mediastinal mass. This was obtained as an inpatient due to the substantial symptoms of joint pain, fevers, and night sweats that she was having. A CT scan of her chest was obtained on May 2, 1998, which demonstrated extensive mediastinal lymphadenopathy, bilateral hilar, as well as upper abdominal lymph nodes. A CT scan of her abdomen obtained on May 6, 1998, demonstrated splenic nodule, as well as porta hepatis and aortocaval lymph nodes. On May 5, 1998, a unilateral bone marrow biopsy was performed to get the diagnosis, and this was negative. A bronchoscopy was also performed which did not yield diagnostic tissue. On May 13, 1998, the biopsy of a left cervical lymph node was performed and established the diagnosis of nodular, sclerosing Hodgkin's disease. Ms. Lieberman's case was discussed with the Multidisciplinary Lymphoma Clinic on May 28, 1998.

Her review of systems is positive for alcohol-induced pruritus, as well as fatigue, fevers, night sweats, weakness, rash, sore throat, shortness of breath, nausea, constipation, stiffness, arthritis, back ache, dizziness, anxiety, and episode of amenorrhea which has resolved with her last menstrual period being May 15, 1998, as well as lump.

Physical exam shows weight 135 pounds, height of 64 inches, temperature 97.8, blood pressure 104/60, and pulse of 77. Her oropharynx is clear with no lesions seen. Chest is clear to auscultation bilaterally. Cardiac exam shows normal S1 and S2 with no murmurs appreciated. Abdominal exam is soft and nontender with no hepatosplenomegaly or masses appreciated. Her nodal exam reveals small, right cervical, left axillary, and left femoral adenopathy, all less than 1 cm. Her extremity exam reveals no edema.

Ms. Lieberman presents to us with stage IIIB nodular, sclerosing Hodgkin's disease. She currently is quite symptomatic with fevers, night sweats, and arthralgias. To this end, she is interested in starting therapy as soon as possible. A MUGA scan was obtained earlier this morning which demonstrates left ventricular ejection fraction of 67%.

We plan to treat Ms. Lieberman with ABVD. This regimen will consist of six 28-day cycles of chemotherapy. The treatment is given on day 1 and day 15 of each cycle. We discussed with Ms. Lieberman the potential and most relevant toxicities of each drug. We discussed the potential for a cardiac injury from the adriamycin. We also mentioned bleomycin can cause pulmonary difficulties, and should a cough or shortness of breath develop, she should contact us. The vinblastine is associated with some peripheral neuropathy, as well as constipation.

We initiated therapy this afternoon with day No. 1 of cycle No. 1. We have given Ms. Lieberman a prescription for Kytril to take over the next three days, as well as a prescription of Ativan and Compazine to help control the nausea. We have also instructed her that should she develop constipation or any other worrisome symptoms, to contact us.

It was a pleasure meeting Ms. Lieberman, and we look forward to keeping you informed of her treatment.

DATE/TIME COLLECTED
  PROCEDURE   RESULT   REFERENCE RANGE

03/30/98 0900
ANTINUCLEAR ANTIBODY: HEP-2
   SCREEN   POSITIVE   *   NEGATIVE
   TITER   1:640   *
   PATTERN   SPECKLED   *

DATE/TIME COLLECTED
  PROCEDURE   RESULT   REFERENCE RANGE

04/29/98 1710
ANTINUCLEAR ANTIBODY: HEP-2
   NAB   POSITIVE   *

NON-FASTING
Recommend anti-dsDNA and anti-ENA if not previously performed
   TITER   1:160   *
)PATTERN   SPECKLED   *

This pattern can be seen in association with a wide variety of autoantibodies
(e.g. anti-ENA). Clinically, many of these individuals have SLE, Sjogren's
syndrome, or MCTD.

ANTINUCLEAR ANTIBODY: HEP-2
   NAB   POSITIVE*
                    05/15/98 1618
                         Recommend anti-dsDNA and anti-ENA if not previously performed
   TITER   1:320*
   PATTERN   SPECKLED*

* = ALPHA ABNORMAL

Labs 4/29/98: White count normal. Hematocrit 34.6 with normal indices and platelets 345,000. Westergren sed rate 69. Urinalysis normal except 6-10 RBC per high power field. Protein was negative 4/30/98. Negative anticardiolipin antibodies, IgG and IgM. Cryoglobulins negative. ANA 1:160 speckled. ANCA negative. ACE within normal limits. CRP 7.1. Serum protein electrophoresis showed increased alpha 1 and 2 globulins and polyclonal gammopathy. CMV and parvo virus B19, IgM antibodies negative. PTT normal at 25.1. DRVVT normal at 33.7. TSH 3.48. T4 total 12.1. ENA 4/2/98 was negative including anti-RNP, Smith, Ro, and La antibodies. C3, C4 normal. DNA negative. ANA on 3/30/98 was 1:640. Rheumatoid factor negative. Lyme antibody negative. Chem panel normal except globulin 3.7 and C02 22.

IMPRESSION:
1) Nodular sclerosing Hodgkin's lymphoma, Stage IIIB, under care of Dr. Erba, with chemotherapy in progress. Involvement includes nodes of the neck region, mediastinum, and involvement of the spleen.
2) Systemic lupus erythematosus with features including:
    a) Positive ANA.
    b) Recurrent oral ulcerations (even proceeding chemotherapy).
    c) Photosensitive rash.
    d) Polyarthralgias/arthritis.
    e) Raynaud's phenomenon.
3) Occasional episodes of tachycardia.
4) Insomnia, occasional depressive symptoms.
5) Small papular skin lesions of fingers and toes, possibly a manifestation of problem #2.
6) Left upper extremity pain in conjunction with port placement.

RECOMMENDATIONS: Unfortunately Ms. Lieberman's arthritic manifestations are sometimes very disabling, confining her at times to a wheelchair.

The patient returns. She carries a diagnosis of nodular sclerosing Hodgkin's lymphoma, Stage IIB, and is receiving chemotherapy, "ABVD" including Adriamycin, bleomycin vincristine, and Decadron. Cough and fever have resolved. She reports a "hollow" sensation in the midsternal region at times.

One major problem has been continued episodes of joint pain and swelling which are controlled when she is on the chemotherapy and rise back up between courses. She did have an additional oral ulceration recently which has resolved. She is not sleeping well at this point and is noticing depressive symptoms occasionally for the first time. She is quite limited by fatigue in terms of activities but has become interested in digital photography using the computer as an alternative activity that she is able to tolerate energy-wise.

Chemo–
   Dr. Erba (friday)

      cycle - 28 days
         treatment every 1st + 15th day
      6 cycles (6 mos) outpatient
      4 drugs ABVD
   lowers blood + marrow count
      WBC - infections, bacteria in blood => hospital, hormone treatment
      RBC - transfusion
      platelets
   side-effects
      fatigue
      nausea, vomitting
      taste
      hair thinning
      weight gain - 5 pounds
      most people dont continue activity
   sick
      2-3 days after treatment
      7-10 days after : fatigue from lowest point WBC
   test
      the A in ABVD weakens heart, muga
      dye in arm to take pic of heart

DURABLE POWER OF ATTORNEY
FOR HEALTH CARE

I, _Jessica Catherine Lieberman_ ,
(Print or type your full name)

am of sound mind, and I voluntarily make this designation.

OPTIONAL

I expressly authorize my patient advocate to make decisions to withhold or withdraw treatment which would allow me to die and I acknowledge such decisions could or would allow my death.

Jessica Lieberman

(Sign your name here if you wish to give your patient advocate this authority.)

Asked about: meds

- circulation (goose bumps)
- rashes (permanet)
- night sweats (recent — used to them)
- nausea, vomiting (no vomitns; nausea a lot — days ago)
- refill one prescription (for nausea?)
- headaches (all the time)
- mouth sores (healing?)
- appetite, weight loss
- chest pain, breath (all the time, but not past wk.)
- fatigue w/ exertion
- light sensitivity
- bowel habits (not good)
- weakness, motor skills (none)
- allergies (e-mysem)
- personal, family med. history
- social history (living here?)

BLEOMYCIN (Injection)

A commonly used brand name is *Blenoxane*.

ABOUT YOUR MEDICINE

Bleomycin (blee-oh-MYE-sin) belongs to the group of medicines called anti-tumor antibiotics. It is used to treat some kinds of cancer.

If any of the information in this leaflet causes you special concern or if you want additional information about your medicine and its use, check with your doctor, nurse, or pharmacist.

out of the reach of children, a

BEFORE USING THIS

Discuss with your doctor the
this medicine. Some of them i

Tell your doctor, nurse, and ph
- are allergic to any medicin
- are pregnant or intend to b
- are breast-feeding;
- are taking any other presc
- have any other medical pr
- have ever been treated wi

PROPER USE OF THI

Bleomycin may often cause
ever, it is very important that
you begin to feel ill. Ask your
these effects.

PRECAUTIONS WHIL

It is very important that your
make sure this medicine is v
fects.

Before you begin using any n
or if you develop any new me
tion, check with your doctor, n

Bleomycin can lower the num
ing the chance of getting an

Special Instructions:

dental or emergency treatment, tell the physician or dentist in charge that you are using this medicine.

POSSIBLE SIDE EFFECTS OF THIS MEDICINE

Side Effects That Should Be Reported To Your Doctor Immediately

---

VINBLASTINE (Injection)

Some commonly used brand names and other names are *Velban*, and *Velsar*, and vinblastine sulfate.

ABOUT YOUR MEDICINE

Vinblastine (vin-BLAS-teen) belongs to the group of medicines known as plant alkaloids. It is used to treat some kinds of cancer as well as some non-cancerous conditions.

If any of the information in this leaflet causes you special concern or if you want additional information a
doctor, nurse, or pharmacist
out of the reach of children, a

BEFORE USING THI

Discuss with your doctor th
this medicine. Some of them

Tell your doctor, nurse, and p
- are allergic to any medici
- are pregnant or intend to
- are breast-feeding;
- are taking any other pres
- have any other medical
  cent exposure), herpes zc
- have ever been treated w

PROPER USE OF TH

While you are using this me
fluids so that you will pass
lems and keep your kidneys

Vinblastine rarely causes na
that you continue to receive
your doctor, nurse, or pharm

PRECAUTIONS WHI

It is very important that you
make sure this medicine is
fects.

Before you begin using any
or if you develop any new m
tion, check with your doctor,

If vinblastine accidentally
it may damage some tiss
nurse right away if you not
injection.

While you are being treated
do not have any immuniza
proval.

Special Instructions:

Vinblastine can lower the number of white blood cells in your blood, increasing the chance of getting an infection. It can also lower the number of platelets, which are necessary for proper blood clotting. If this occurs:
- Avoid people with infections.
- Be careful when using a regular toothbrush, dental floss, or toothpick.

DACARBAZINE (Injection)

A commonly used brand name is *DTIC-Dome*.

ABOUT YOUR MEDICINE

Dacarbazine (da-KAR-ba-zeen) belongs to the group of medicines called alkylating agents. It is used to treat some kinds of cancer.

If any of the information in this leaflet causes you special concern or if you want additional information about your medicine and its use, check with your doctor, nurse, or pharmacist
out of the reach of children,

BEFORE USING THI

Discuss with your doctor th
this medicine. Some of them

Tell your doctor, nurse, and
- are allergic to any medici
- are pregnant or intend to
- are breast-feeding;
- are taking any other pres
- have any other medica
  recent exposure), herpe
  or liver disease;
- have ever been treated w

PROPER USE OF TH

This medicine often causes
jection may also cause a fe
portant that you continue
discomfort or begin to feel l
lessen. Ask your doctor, nu
fects.

PRECAUTIONS WHI

It is very important that you
make sure this medicine is
fects.

Before you begin using any
or if you develop any new m
tion, check with your doctor,

While you are being treated
do not have any immuniza
proval.

Special Instructions:

Dacarbazine can lower the number of white blood cells in your blood, increasing the chance of getting an infection. It can also lower the number of platelets, which are necessary for proper blood clotting. If this occurs:
- Avoid people with infections.
- Be careful when using a regular toothbrush, dental floss, or toothpick.

PARTNERS IN HEALTH
Hemotology/Oncology Outpatient Services

ADRIAMYCIN
(Adria, Doxorubicin, Hydroxyl daunorubicin)

USE

A chemotherapy drug given intravenously to fight cancer cells.

SPECIAL INSTRUCTIONS

Tissue damage may occur at the needle insertion site if the medication leaks out of the vein. If youfeel any burning and/or pain at the needle insertion site or traveling up the arm, notify the nurse immediately.

PRECAUTIONS

Should you have any unusual bleeding, signs of infection or a temperature of 100.5 or above, notify your doctor or nurse immediately or come directly to the Emergency Room.

SIDE EFFECTS

Early Side Effects

Nausea, vomiting and diarrhea may occur within one to two hours after administration and last for 24 hours. You will receive medication to help prevent this problem 1/2 hour before receiving the drug.

Pink to red-orange urine may occur for 1-3 days after receiving Adriamycin due to its red color. This is normal and not a cause for concern.

Late Side Effects

Bone Marrow Suppression is a decrease in the number of white blood cells, red blood cells, and platelets, predisposing you to infections, anemia, or bleeding problems.

Hair Loss occurs in most patients. See information regarding U of M Wig Bank.

-1-

Department of Internal Medicine
University of Michigan Medical Center

Radiology and Nuclear Medicine Results

Status	**Requisition Number**	**Date**	**Source System**
F	1755449	6/12/1998	RIS

PORT PLACEMENT

CLINICAL INFORMATION:

HODGKIN'S. NEED FOR LONG-TERM TREATMENT.

PROCEDURE:

Following explanation of the risks, benefits, and alternatives
informed oral and written consent was obtained for port placement.

The left arm was prepped and draped observing surgical scrub
technique. Operator's observed surgical scrub. Under fluoroscopic
observation, 20 cc Omnipaque 240 was injected through a peripheral IV
and the left basilic vein punctured with a micropuncture set.
Following local anesthesia with lidocaine with epinephrine, a
subcutaneous pocket was created by blunt dissection. The catheter was
sized and attached to the port. The port was placed in the pocket and
secured with absorbable suture. The catheter was delivered through a
peel-away sheath and its tip positioned in the central superior vena
cava. The incision was closed in two layers. Skin sutures may be
removed in ten days.

There were no immediate complications.

Medications: 2 mg Versed, 100 ugm Fentanyl.

Primary operator - Dr. Orsinelli.
Teaching staff - Dr. David Williams, who was present for the critical
portion of the procedure.

IMPRESSION:

1. Successful placement of S-port via left basilic vein. Tip in
central superior vena cava.

CHEMOTHEREAPY DIARY

DATE	VISIT/CALL	SYMPTOMS
May 29	Treatment 1	
May 30		fatigue
May 31		fatigue, constipation
June 1	7am Cancer Center for severe constipation: anema (diarrhea for rest of day)	
June 2	4pm Cancer Center for blurred vision, loopiness/dizziness, slurred words (start last night)- Dr. Erba decided problem was likely Compazine, which I stopped taking, problem solved	
June 3		diarrhea
June 4		
June 5		
June 6		fatigue, p.m. Joint pain
June 7		Joint Pain, mouth irritation and pain, bleeding anus
June 8		milder joint pain, mouth irritation (tarry stool?) Depression (?)
June 9		severe ankle pain (L), regular joint pain (ankle, knees, wrist)
June 10		severe ankle pain (L) and lower back pain
June 11		severe ankle pain (L) and joint pain

DATE	VISIT/CALL	SYMPTOMS
Fri June 12	Port Placement Treatment 2	severe ankle pain
Sat June 13		am nausea, bad cramping and constipation, Lactulose @ 4pm relief ~ 3 hours later, then diarrhea for rest of night
		icky metal taste in mouth
		port wound bled and oozed through three bandages of steri-strips and gauze through to ace bandage
	12 p.m. called Radiologist on call about oozing, he said it was not normal and to go to ER, I tried Cancer Center which was closed and then did not go to ER (too scared to deal)	
Sun June 14		arm seems better but hurts, fatigue, diarrhea Depression
Mon June 15		a.m. fever (no thermometer), fatigue and discomfort during walk in sun, severe headaches throughout day, very tired, much mouth irritation, mouth pain, big white sore, some throat pain, diarrhea, and pain in ears- BAD DAY
	6:30 called Hem on call about mouth sore, she wasn't worried	
		couldn't eat dinner, mouth hurt too much Depression and nightmares/ stress dreams
Tues June 16		woke feeling horrible, mouth pain and upper stomach/lower chest pain (hollowness, acidic) and general yuckiness, walk made me clammy and very fatigued, couldn't eat until 5pm
Wed June 17		woke at 5 am extremely tense, grinding teeth and stressed some ankle pain (L) and mouth pain but not as bad fatigue and discomfort in upper stomach area but not as bad

Thur June 18		Fatigue
Fri June 19		first normal poop, Arm Pain still wont go away (isn't it time?)
Sat June 20		normal poop!, Tingling in finger tips on left hand, numbish as if asleep, arm is still very swollen and painful from wrist to armpit
Sun June 21		normal poop!! Same arm and finger problems
M June 22		
T June 23		
W June 24		Appt. with Kazmers- diagnosis of Lupus, prescription of Prednisone and Plaquinil
T June 25		

F Jun 26	Treatment	
S Jun 27		begin Prednisone (5) and Plaquinil

Chemotherapy
Pre-Meds:

Kytril	1mg	oral
Ativan	1 mg	oral
Decadron	20 mg	IV
Tylenol	650 mg	oral

Chemo meds:

Adria	41 mg	IV
Velban	9.9 mg	IV
Bleomyocin	16.5 mg	IV
Dar	615 mg	IV

Please Place **USED** Nipple Markers On This Sheet.

Not For Reuse

We had the pleasure of seeing Jessica Lieberman in the Hematology Clinic

As you know, she is a 27-year-old woman with stage IIIB nodular sclerosis Hodgkin s disease.

blood pressure 99/58; heart rate 83; respiratory rate 16; and temperature 96.5. HEENT exam is unremarkable.

Her hair has started to come back. Her sclerae are anicteric. Extraocular movements are intact. Oropharynx is clear. Her neck is supple without thyromegaly. Her lungs are clear bilaterally. There are no wheezes or crackles. There are no pleural rubs. Cardiac exam shows a regular rate and rhythm, without any murmurs, rubs, or gallops. Her abdomen is soft, nontender, and nondistended, without any organomegaly. Examination of her lymph node groups shows no cervical, axillary, supraclavicular, or inguinal adenopathy.

The only notable finding on exam is her skin. She has some mild erythema in the area of her mantle field, most prominent superiorly. There is no desquamation. There is no hyperpigmentation. She also has some erythema in the area of her spade field.

Plan: Prednisone 15 mg p.o. q.a.m. for the next two to four weeks. A return visit is suggested in one month. Labs and serologies will be updated today including urinalysis, ANA, ANA subtypes, and complement levels.

I appreciate the opportunity to see Ms. Lieberman.

The patient continues to receive chemotherapy for nodular sclerosing Hodgkin's lymphoma stage IIIB at University of Michigan Medical Center. She has developed alopecia secondary to this as well as generalized tiredness and decreased exercise tolerance. The patient is noticing an accentuation of photosensitivity with redness of the face and swelling of the hands, pain in the hands, and accentuated fatigue with sun exposure. She does use a sun blocker and protective clothing when she goes out but avoids staying outside for any length of time because of this.

This is a new patient. This is a 27-year-old white female here for evaluation of a rash that she developed two days ago. The patient has a past medical history of systemic lupus erythematosus and nodular sclerosing Hodgkin's disease. The patient says she was diagnosed with both of these disorders in late May\early June.

Social History: The patient is a grad student working on her doctorate in english.

Physical Examination: The patient's face, neck, chest, arms and legs examined. The patient with macular erythema of the face, upper chest and back. It also extends onto the arms where there is a slight papular component. The erythema is significantly more prominent on the upper half of the body as compared to the lower half. The patient has only areas of involvement of her lower torso and legs. There is no scale or other surface changes to this rash and the patient does find it quite itchy and she is scratching it in the office this morning.

66

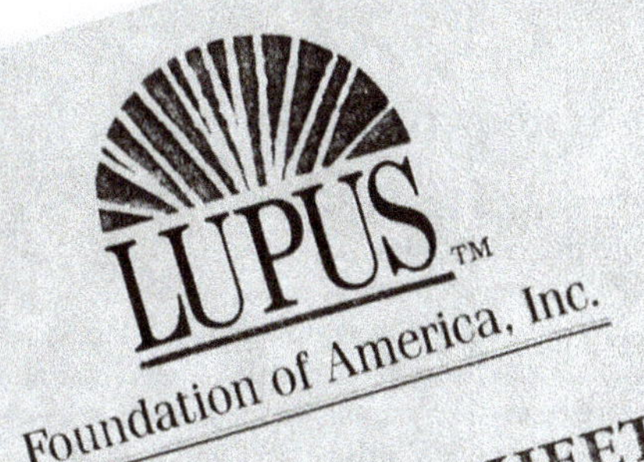

Foundation of America, Inc.

LUPUS FACT SHEET

- Lupus is a chronic, autoimmune disease which causes inflammation of various parts of the body, especially the skin, joints, blood and kidneys. The immune system normally protects the body against viruses, bacteria and other foreign materials. In an autoimmune disease like lupus, the immune system loses its ability to tell the difference between foreign substances and its own cells and tissues. The immune system then makes antibodies directed against itself.

- Lupus is NOT infectious, rare or cancerous.

- LFA market research data show that between 1,400,000 and 2,000,000 people have been diagnosed with lupus. (Study conducted by Bruskin/Goldring Research.) Lupus is more widespread than AIDS, sickle cell anemia, cerebral palsy, multiple sclerosis and cystic fibrosis combined.

- Although the cause of lupus is unknown, scientists suspect that individuals are genetically predisposed to lupus, and know that environmental factors such as infections, antibiotics, ultraviolet light, extreme stress and certain drugs play a critical role in triggering the disease.

- Lupus affects 1 out of every 185 Americans. Although lupus can strike men and women of all ages, 90% of people with lupus are women and during the childbearing years. Lupus is more prevalent (3 times more frequently) than men. Lupus is more prevalent among black, Hispanic, Native Americans and Asians.

- Only 10% of people with lupus will have a close relative (parent or sibling) who already has or may develop lupus. Only about 5% of the children born to individuals with lupus will develop the illness.

- Lupus can be difficult to diagnose as the symptoms come and go and mimic those of other diseases. Some symptoms of lupus can be transient joint and muscle pain, weakness, extreme fatigue, hair loss, photosensitivity, low grade fevers. Some symptoms worsen by sunlight, painful sensitivity of the fingers to the cold.

- Sunlight, infection, injury, surgery, stress or exhaustion may bring on symptoms or cause a "flare" (active state of the disease).

- Although lupus ranges from mild to life-threatening and thousands of Americans die of lupus each year, the majority of cases can be controlled with proper treatment.

- Increased professional awareness and improved diagnostic techniques and evaluation methods are contributing to the early diagnosis and treatment of lupus. With current methods of therapy, 80-90% of people with lupus can look forward to a normal lifespan.

- While medical science has not yet developed a method for curing lupus, new research brings unexpected findings and increased hope each year.

- The Lupus Foundation of America has nearly 100 local chapters directly providing patient services, education, awareness and research in their local areas.

2-95

4 Research Place, Suite 180, Rockville, MD 20850-3226 (301) 670-9292 • (800) 558-0121

OUT-PATIENT NOTES

DATE 6-22-98   DIAGNOSIS HODGKIN'S DISEASE

WT 130   KARNOFSKY SCORE ____

MCARE GRAD CARE   OUT
F 06 07 71 ANN ARBOR
LIEBERMAN, JESSICA
02749 742 1
VISIT

INTERIM HISTORY 978 90/50 93
day II cycle Ib ABVD

c/o persistent ① arm pain since port placed.
unable to extend ① elbow
paresthesia ① 2,3,4th fingertip

①H/C

med: inc. coumadin 5 mg qd

PHYSICAL

tender to palpation ① upper arm and medial forearm to wrist
minimal swelling ① upper arm
no edema ① hand.
no sig erythema
no d/c from surgical wound

CHEMOTHERAPY   062298

HGB ____   HEMAT ____
WBC ____   PLATS ____
DIFF-SEG ____ BAND ____ LYMPH ____
MONO ____ EO ____ BASO ____ BLAST ____
OTHER ____

PBS REVIEWED: YES NO
FINDINGS:
INTERPRETATION:

NURSING/CHEMOTHERAPY NOTE

X-RAYS Doppler U/S ① UE – no evidence for DVT

IMPRESSION

PROGRAM (RV with STUDIES) Refer to Angio for suture removal and assessment

LETTER YES ____ NO ____

HARRY ERBA, MD
ATTENDING STAFF

HEMATOLOGY/ONCOLOGY

CONSULTATION

DATE: 11-19-98

REFERRING PHYSICIAN: Harry Erba, M.D., Division of Hematology Oncology

DIAGNOSIS: Stage IIIB nodular sclerosing Hodgkin's disease.

HISTORY OF PRESENT ILLNESS: Jessica Lieberman is a 27-year-old female who was doing well until March 2, 1998 when she developed some left groin pain which awakened her. She subsequently developed arthralgias, skin excoriations, photosensity, rash, and Raynaud's syndrome. She was then evaluated on March 23rd by her primary care physician for possible Lyme disease, who then started her on Indocin for pain control. This, however, had little effect and the patient additionally developed left-sided chest pain, anorexia, fatigue, fevers to 101°, chills, and drenching night sweats. Given the history of the chest pain and cough, a chest x-ray was obtained and read as having mediastinal plus hilar adenopathy, which is believed to be either secondary to lymphoma or granulomatous disease. She was then admitted to the Rheumatology Service from May 1st through the 4th for a work-up. A CT done at that time showed mediastinal and hilar adenopathy, as well as a low attenuation lesion in the spleen. Small paraortic lymph nodes were also present, but no other pathology was noted. Given the lymphadenopathy a transbronchial biopsy was performed, but was non-diagnostic. Rheum evaluation, however, at that time showed a positive ANA ratio of 1:640 and a sed rate elevated to 66. A bone marrow biopsy was performed additionally at that time and showed trilinear hematopoiesis and no lymphoma. A photocytometry also was negative for lymphoma and leukemia. The patient was then sent to General Surgery for a lymph node biopsy from a low left cervical node, and path from this revealed the nodular sclerosing Hodgkin's disease. A staging CT was then done and showed mediastinal disease, including the right paratracheal subcarinal and hilar regions, as well as celiac and portal hepatic adenopathy. The small abnormality in the spleen was again noted, but there was otherwise no evidence of abdominal or pelvic adenopathy. During this whole period, her fevers and night sweats persisted, but her weight remained stable. Her symptoms of rash and groin pain also persisted. She was at that time seen by Dr. Lichter and Dr. Dornfeld in Radiation Oncology, who felt that chemotherapy would be appropriate.

Dr. Erba, who started ABVD chemo on 06-03-98, then saw the patient. She tolerated this well. A CT done on September 11th revealed a decrease in size of the low-attenuation lesion in the spleen, and made it likely that this was also involved in the Hodgkin's disease. It also showed a 90% decrease in the thoracic lymphadenopathy, most notably in the mediastinal and paratracheal regions. As such, in September, after 4 cycles, she was classified as having a complete remission. She continued to have 2 more cycles through the end of October, and a CT following the final cycle revealed no adenopathy and no changes compared to the September scan. Dr. Erba, who recommended that radiation therapy could potentially decrease the relapse rate, but not change the overall survival, then saw her. She presents here to Dr. Lichter again, for possible radiation therapy.

In regards to symptoms, she continues to note occasional chills, but is otherwise without any B-symptoms of fevers, night sweats, or weight loss. She has not noted any new masses or lymph node enlargement anywhere.

PAST MEDICAL HISTORY:

1) Guillain Barre's-type disease which the patient developed at around the age of 12, but which has not caused any further problems.

2) Possible TMJ.

3) Systemic lupus erythematosus, which was diagnosed secondary to the patient having a rash, as well as migrating arthralgias. As these symptoms, as well as the elevated ANA had persisted through the chemotherapy, they were believed secondary to his collagen vascular disease and not due to the Hodgkin's.

PHYSICAL EXAMINATION: Ms. Lieberman is alert and oriented times 3 and in no acute distress. HEENT: PERRLA, EOMI, sclera anicteric, no nasal discharge, audition intact, neck supple. Oral mucosa reveals 2 to 3 very small lesions on the anterior hard palate which are healing well. There is otherwise no evidence of any erythema or exudate on the oropharynx. A very small 0.5 cm to 1 cm lymph node is palpable in the anterocervical region on the right side. There is otherwise no cervical, supraclavicular, axillary, or inguinal adenopathy. Chest is clear to auscultation, with no rhonchi, rales, or wheezing bilaterally. Cardiac exam reveals a regular rate and rhythm, regular S1, S2, and no murmurs. There is no pain to palpation of the spine or back. Abdomen is soft, nontender, and nondistended, with positive bowel sounds. No organomegaly or masses could be appreciated. Extremities are without clubbing, cyanosis, or edema. On neurologic exam, cranial nerves II-XII are intact, and there is no evidence of any focal, motor, sensory, or cerebellar signs. Skin exam reveals some slightly erythematous, raised patch-like rashes over the anterior chest, and posterior neck. These reportedly have been there for quite some time by the patient.

RADIOLOGIC DATA:

1) CT of chest 05-02-98: Bilateral hilar and extensive mediastinal lymph node enlargement and enlarged upper abdominal lymph nodes. Most notably are those in the anterior mediastinum, right paratracheal, subcarinal, and hilar lymph node grooves. There are also enlarged lymph nodes in the celiac and portal hepatic region. There is also a 1 cm low-attenuation abnormality in the posterior aspect of the spleen.

IMPRESSION: Jessica Lieberman is a 27-year-old with newly diagnosed stage IIIB nodular sclerosing Hodgkin's disease status-post ABVD chemotherapy, now here for possible radiation therapy.

RECOMMENDATIONS: The patient's current situation was discussed extensively with her, as well as to friends who are present. She was informed that Hodgkin's patients receiving radiation therapy, although they did have a decreased relapse rate of roughly 30% to 15%, did not have an overall increased survival rate. Additionally, it was noted that patients who have had radiation therapy tend to do worse on chemotherapy for relapse. She was also informed that having radiation would increase the risk of a second malignancy in the radiation field, including such things as breast cancer and thyroid cancer. Additionally, a concern was expressed regarding the use of the low-dose radiation and the patient's diagnosis of lupus, but the significance of this has yet to be determined. She was told to make her decision regardless of the lupus, and was told either to receive radiation or not to is a reasonable option. It is highly possible that this patient is cured and requires no further therapy, but it is difficult to tell at this time. She will ask Dr. Erba for his personal opinion, but we feel at this time that radiation therapy would be useful. She has received all the information and will discuss the case with her father, who is a physician, and will return with her decision shortly. In the interim, we would also like to make sure that the patient has a gallium scan, as a positive scan would alter her potential options for therapy. Additionally, inquiries will be made as to the interaction between low-dose radiation and patients with lupus. She was told that radiation therapy would consist of 10 treatments, half to the anterior mediastinum and chest and the other half to the abdomen, and it could be done upon returning from her Christmas vacation on January 5th if necessary.

POSSIBLE SIDE EFFECTS OF THIS MEDICINE

Side Effects That Should Be Reported To Your Doctor Immediately

Less common—Cough or hoarseness; fever or chills; lower back or side pain; painful or difficult urination; redness, pain, or swelling at place of injection

Rare—Black, tarry stools; blood in urine or stools; pinpoint red spots on skin; unusual bleeding or bruising

Other Side Effects That Should Be Reported To Your Doctor

Less common—Joint pain; sores in mouth and on lips; swelling of feet or lower legs

Rare—Difficulty in walking; dizziness; double vision; drooping eyelids; headache; jaw pain; mental depression; numbness or tingling in fingers and toes; pain in fingers and toes; pain in testicles; weakness

Side Effects That Usually Do Not Require Medical Attention

These possible side effects may go away during treatment; however, if they continue or are bothersome, check with your doctor, nurse, or pharmacist.

Less common—Muscle pain; nausea and vomiting

This medicine often causes a temporary loss of hair. After treatment with vinblastine has ended, or sometimes even during treatment, normal hair growth should return.

Other side effects not listed above may also occur in some patients. If you notice any other effects, check with your doctor, nurse, or pharmacist.

The information in this leaflet has been selectively abstracted from USP DI for use as an educational aid and does not cover all possible uses, actions, precautions, side effects, or interactions of this medicine. It is not intended as medical advice for individual problems.

Hair Loss occurs in most patients. See information regarding U of M Wig Bank.

ALLERGIES / SENSITIVITIES: To prednisone which caused nausea and vomiting.

DIET: Regular.

ACTIVITY: As tolerated.

CONDITION OF PATIENT AT DISCHARGE: Alive.

MEDICATION:
CEVIMELINE HCL 30 MG CAPSULE, #60505-3145-01

IMPORTANT:
HOW TO USE THIS INFORMATION: THIS IS A SUM
ABOUT THIS PRODUCT.

COMMON BRAND NAME(S):
Evoxac

USES:
This medication is used to treat symptoms of dry mouth du
to a class of drugs known as cholinergic agonists. It wo
produce, making it easier and more comfortable to speak a

HOW TO USE:
Take this medication by mouth with or without food, usual
medical condition and response to treatment.   Use this me
take it at the same times each day.   You may continue to d
You may start to feel some benefit in 1 to 2 weeks. Howev
your condition persists or worsens.

SIDE EFFECTS:
See also Precautions.   Sweating, nausea, runny nose, flusl
vision may occur. If any of these effects persist or worsen,
increase in tears. This can be helpful if you have dry eyes.
doctor has prescribed this medication because he or she h
Many people using this medication do not have serious s
serious side effects occur: slow/fast/irregular heartbe
wheezing/cough/phlegm), mental/mood changes (such as
allergic reaction to this drug is rare. However, seek imme

NONSTEROIDAL ANTI-INFLAMMATORY DRUGS -

ES: Also known as NSAIDs, this medication relieve
duces inflammation. It is used to treat headaches,
hes, dental pain, menstrual cramps and athletic ir
commonly used to treat pain, swelling and stiffne
th arthritis. This medication can also reduce feve

W TO TAKE THIS MEDICATION: If stomach upset occur
is medication, take it with food, milk or an antac
dication is most effective in relieving menstrual
the earliest sign of pain.

DE EFFECTS: Stomach upset is the most common side
is persists or becomes severe, notify your doctor.
Inform your doctor if you develop persistent stom
esence of black or bloody stools, skin rash, itchi
welling of the feet or hands), change in urine col
anges while taking this medication.
May cause dizziness, drowsiness or blurred vision. Avoid
tivities requiring alertness if this occurs. May rarely cause
nging in the ears and or loss of hearing.
Infrequently, this medication may increase the skin's
nsitivity to sunlight. If this happens to you, avoid prolonged
n exposure, wear protective clothing and use a sun
nlamps.

ECAUTIONS: Tell your doctor your medical history
y liver or kidney disease, blood disorders, ulcers
sease, alcohol use, high blood pressure, eye disea
lergies, especially drug allergies.
Use caution when performing tasks requiring alert
cohol intake as it may intensify the drowsiness ef
dication and make your stomach or intestines more
eed.
Do not take aspirin without co
e ingredients of any nonprescri
king since many cough and cold

MEDICATION:
HYDROCODON-ACETAMINOPH 7.5-325, #00603-3891-21

IMPORTANT:
HOW TO USE THIS INFORMATION: THIS IS A SUMMARY AND DOES NOT HAVE ALL POSSIBLE
ABOUT THIS PRODUCT.

COMMON BRAND NAME(S):
Lorcet, Lortab, Norco, Vicodin

WARNING:
One ingredient in this product is acetaminophen. Taking too much acetaminophen may cause serious (possibly f
Adults should not take more than 4000 milligrams (4 grams) of acetaminophen a day. If you have liver proble
doctor or pharmacist for a safe dosage of this medication. Daily use of alcohol, especially when combined with ace
increase your risk for liver damage. Avoid alcohol. Check with your doctor or pharmacist for more information.
right away if you have any symptoms of liver damage, including: dark urine, persistent nausea/vomiting, stomach/abdominal pain,
extreme tiredness, or yellowing eyes/skin.   Acetaminophen is an ingredient found in many nonprescription products and in some
combination prescription medications (such as pain/fever drugs or cough-and-cold products). Carefully check the labels on all your
medicines because they may also contain acetaminophen. Ask your pharmacist about using those products safely. Get medical help
right away if you have taken more than 4000 milligrams of acetaminophen a day, even if you feel well.

USES:
This combination medication is used to relieve moderate to severe pain. It contains a narcotic pain reliever (hydrocodone) and a non-
narcotic pain reliever (acetaminophen). Hydrocodone works in the brain to change how your body feels and responds to pain.
Acetaminophen can also reduce a fever.

HOW TO USE:
See also Warning section.   Read the Patient Information Leaflet if available from your pharmacist before you start taking this
medication and each time you get a refill. If you have any questions, ask your doctor or pharmacist.   Take this medication by mouth
as directed by your doctor. You may take this drug with or without food. If you have nausea, it may help to take this drug with food.
Ask your doctor or pharmacist about other ways to decrease nausea (such as lying down for 1 to 2 hours with as little head
movement as possible).   If you are using a liquid form of this medication, use a medication measuring device to carefully measure
the prescribed dose. Do not use a household spoon because you may not get the correct dose.   The dosage is based on your medical
condition and response to treatment. In children, the dosage is also based on weight. Do not increase your dose, take the medication
more frequently, or take it for a longer time than prescribed. Properly stop the medication when so directed.   Pain medications work
best if they are used as the first signs of pain occur. If you wait until the pain has worsened, the medication may not work as well.
If you have ongoing pain (such as due to cancer), your doctor may direct you to also take long-acting narcotic medications. In that
case, this medication might be used for sudden (breakthrough) pain only as needed. Other non-narcotic pain relievers (such as
naproxen, ibuprofen) may also be prescribed with this medication. Ask your doctor or pharmacist if you have any questions about
using this product safely with other drugs.   This medication may cause withdrawal reactions, especially if it has been used regularly
for a long time or in high doses. In such cases, withdrawal symptoms (such as restlessness, watering eyes, runny nose, nausea,
sweating, muscle aches) may occur if you suddenly stop using this medication. To prevent withdrawal reactions, your doctor may
reduce your dose gradually. Ask your doctor or pharmacist for more details, and report any withdrawal reactions immediately.

PROCHLORPERAZINE

(proe klor per' a zeen)

OTHER NAME : Compazine

WHY is this drug prescribed?
Prochlorperazine controls the nausea and vomiting caused by radiation
therapy, cancer chemotherapy, surgery, and various conditions. It is also
used to treat psychotic symptoms such as hallucinations and hostility.

WHEN should it be used?
Prochlorperazine usually is taken three or four times a day
(controlled-release capsules are taken once or twice a day). Follow the
instructions on your prescription label carefully, and ask your pharmacis
or doctor to explain any part that you do not understand.
Prochlorperazine starts to work in about 30 to 40 minutes (60 minutes whe
taken rectally) and goes on working for three to four hours (10 to 12
hours for controlled-release capsules). Although prochlorperazine is not
habit-forming, do not stop taking it abruptly, especially if you have bee
taking it for a long time. Your doctor probably will want to decrease you
dose gradually.

HOW should it be used?
Prochlorperazine comes in tablets, cont
capsules, oral liquid, and rectal suppo
tells you how much prochlorperazine to
controlled-release capsules; swallow tl
specially marked measuring spoon from
accurate dose of the liquid. Do not al
it can cause irritation.
To insert a rectal suppository, follow
feels soft, hold it under cold, running
the wrapper. 2. Dip the tip of the supp
your left side and raise your right kne
person should lie on the right side and
your finger, insert the suppository int
in children and 1 inch in adults. Hold
moments. 5. Stand up after about 15 min
and resume your normal activities. Ask
have about refilling your prescription.

What SPECIAL INSTRUCTIONS should I foll
Prochlorperazine can cause drowsiness.
dangerous machinery until you know how
to the drowsiness caused by prochlorpe
alcoholic beverages. Keep all appointme
need to be adjusted occasionally, espec
drug. You also should have eye examinat
prochlorperazine for a long time. Be sv
this medication on hand. Check your sup
other occasions you may not be able to

What should I do IF I FORGET to take a
Take the missed dose as soon as you rer
doses for that day at evenly spaced int
missed dose at the time you are schedul
the regularly scheduled one. Do not tak

MEDICATION:
CLINDAMYCIN HCL 150 MG CAPSULE, #65862-0185-0

IMPORTANT:
HOW TO USE THIS INFORMATION: THIS IS A SUMI
ABOUT THIS PRODUCT.

COMMON BRAND NAME(S):
Cleocin

WARNING:

MEDICATION:
CHLORHEXIDINE 0.12% RINSE, #00116-2001-16

IMPORTANT:
HOW TO USE THIS INFORMATION: THIS IS A
ABOUT THIS PRODUCT.

COMMON BRAND NAME(S):
Peridex, Periogard

USES:
This medication is used along with regular tooth bru
easily bleeding gums. Chlorhexidine belongs to a c
bacteria in the mouth, helping to reduce swelling and

OTHER USES:
This section contains uses of this drug that are no
prescribed by your health care professional. Use thi
by your health care professional.   Chlorhexidine i
formation of mouth sores (mucositis), and used to he

HOW TO USE:
Rinse your mouth with the solution after brushing
your doctor. M
for 30 seconds, a
at least 30 minu
on your medical
remember, use it
doctor if your c

SIDE EFFECT
Tooth/tongue sta
persist or worsen
3 times daily, br
See your dentist
work (such as cr
first, followed by
because he or she
notice any symp
face/tongue/thro
effects not listed
You may report

USES: Loratadine is an antihistamine that provides relief of
symptoms of seasonal and allergic rhinitis such as watery eyes,
runny nose, itching eyes and sneezing. It is also used for hives.

ION: Take this medication by mouth once a

dose or take this more often than

cation for several days before allergy
ts can be affected.

cation may cause headache, thirst, blurred
y nose. These effects should subside as
medication. If they continue or become

MEDICATION:
LEVOTHYROXINE 100 MCG TABLET, #00781-5184-92

IMPORTANT:
HOW TO USE THIS INFORMATION: THIS IS A SUMMARY AND D
ABOUT THIS PRODUCT.

COMMON BRAND NAME(S):
Levothroid, Levoxyl, Synthroid, Unithroid

WARNING:
This medication should not be used for weight loss. Normal doses of this m
of this medication may cause serious, possibly fatal side effects, especially w

USES:
Levothyroxine is used to treat an underactive thyroid (hypothyroidism). It
normally produced by the thyroid gland. Low thyroid hormone levels can
radiation/medications or removed by surgery. Having enough thyroid horm
physical activity. In children, having enough thyroid hormone is important
medication is also used to treat other types of thyroid disorders (such as cer
should not be used to treat infertility unless it is caused by low thyroid horm

HOW TO USE:
Take this medication by mouth as directed by your doctor, usually once da
breakfast. Take this medication with a full glass of water unless your doct
form of this medication, swallow it whole. Do not split, crush, or chew.
infants or small children) should use the tablet form of the medication.   Fc
crush the tablet and mix in 1 to 2 teaspoons (5 to 10 milliliters) of water, a
prepare a supply in advance or mix the tablet in soy infant formula. Cons
based on your age, weight, medical condition, laboratory test results, and r

CORTICOSTEROIDS - TOPICAL

USES: This medication is used to treat swelling, inflammation,
or itching of skin conditions such as eczema, dermatitis, rashe
insect bites, poison ivy, allergies and other irritations.

HOW TO USE THIS MEDICATION: Clean and dry the affected area
before applying the medication.
   To apply, gently massage a small amount of the medication in
the affected area and surrounding skin.
   Cover with a bandage only if instructed to do so by your doc
Do not use plastic pants or tight fitting diapers on children
being treated with this medication in the diaper area.
Some bandages and covering can increase the effects of this
medication resulting in side effects.
   Avoid using this medication around the eyes unless directed
do so by your doctor.

SIDE EFFECTS: This medication may cause burning, stinging,
itching or redness when first applied to the skin. This should
disappear in a few days as your body adjusts to the medication.
If these effects persist or worsen, inform your doctor.
   Skin infections can become worse when using this medication.
Notify your doctor if redness, swelling or irritation does not
improve.

PRECAUTIONS: Do not use this medication near the eyes if you h
glaucoma.
   Treatment with alclometasone, clobetasol, halobetasol
propionate and augmented betamethasone dipropionate beyond two
weeks consecutively is not recommended.
   Do not use if there is an infection or sores present on the
area to be treated.
   This medication should be used cautiously during pregnancy a
only if clearly needed. Discuss the benefits and risks with you
doctor. Small amounts of this medication may appear in breast
milk. Consult with your doctor before breast-feeding.

directed by your doctor. Take it
Do not lie down for at least 10
se to treatment. In children, the
ody is kept at a constant level.
ll prescribed amount is finished,
turn of the infection.   Tell your

ist or worsen, tell your doctor
he has judged that the benefit to
s side effects.   Tell your doctor
ely if any of these rare but very
amount of urine.   Use of this
ction. Contact your doctor if you

INDOMETHACIN - ORAL CAPSULE, TABLET

USES: This medication relieves pain and reduces inflammation. It is commonly used to treat pain, swelling and stiffness associated with arthritis, gout, bursitis and tendonitis.

ABOUT YOUR MEDICINE
   GRANISETRON (gra-NI-se-tron) is used to prevent the nausea and vomiting that may occur after treatment with anticancer medicines (chemotherapy).
   If any of the information in this leaflet causes you special concern or if you want additional information about your medicine and its use, check with your doctor, nurse, or pharmacist. REMEMBER, KEEP THIS AND ALL OTHER MEDICINES OUT OF THE REACH OF CHILDREN AND NEVER SHARE YOUR MEDICINES WITH OTHERS.

IS MEDICINE
ctor, nurse, and pharmacist if you . . .
ic to any medicine, either prescription or
ption (OTC);
nt or intend to become pregnant;
-feeding
 any other prescription or nonprescription (OTC)

ther medical problems.

LE USING THIS MEDICINE
our doctor if you have severe nausea and vomiting after
therapy.

1 or immediately after
 full glass of water.
:ions must be swallowed
:ained activity may

mmon side effect. If
: doctor.
ightheadedness,
 or nervousness may
1.
:ent stomach pain,
3h, itching, edema
:hanges while taking

SIBLE INFORMATION

ight loss, and large doses

OMEPRAZOLE - ORAL SUSTAINED RELEASE CAPSULE

is medication works by reducing the amount of acid
by the stomach. It is used in the treatment of conditions
phageal reflux disease, in the treatment of conditions
ne Zollinger-Ellison Syndrome where excessive stomach
roduced, and in the treatment of erosive esophagitis.
istances, this medication may be prescribed for treatmen
al or gastric (stomach) ulcers, alone or added to
es to help cure ulcers related to infection (H pylori).

KE THIS MEDICATION: This medication works best if taken
ting. Antacids may be taken with this medication.
psules are sustained-release and must be swallowed whole
ush or chew them or the long action may be destroyed and
e of side effects increased.

CTS: This medication may cause diarrhea, constipation,
che, nausea, gas, loss of appetite, headache or
 the first few days as your body adjusts to it. If these
ersist or become bothersome, inform your doctor.
ly but tell your doctor if you develop a skin rash, back
pain, nervousness, sleep disturbances, cough or chest
hing, breathing trouble, swelling of the hands or feet,
hirst, change in amount of urine or
edication may rarely cause loss of b
lling of stomach or fatigue.

NS: Tell your doctor if you have li

yroid hormone, which is
yroid gland is injured by
ning normal mental and
sical development. This
ancer). This medication

minutes to 1 hour before
ou are taking the capsule
e capsule whole (such as
pper immediately. Do not
information. Dosage is
is medication regularly in
p taking this medication
re are different brands of
   Certain medications
nate, calcium carbonate,
y of these drugs, separate
tiredness, muscle aches,
n worsens or persists after

our body adjusts to this
our doctor has prescribed
. Many people using this

CORTICOSTEROIDS - ORAL

USES: This medication belongs to a class of drugs
corticosteroids. Corticosteroids have various effe
They reduce swelling and inflammation. Corticoster
a variety of disorders such as skin diseases (psor
allergic conditions, asthma, respiratory condition
blood disorders (anemia), digestive problems, eye
rheumatic disorders (arthritis, bursitis) and repl
adrenal gland hormones.

HOW TO TAKE T
a meal to pre
   Take this
carefully. Be
   If you are
taken in the
   The liquid
   If you hav
suddenly stop
may need to b
fatigue, weak
is suddenly s

SIDE EFFECTS:
increased app
These effects
medication. I
doctor.
   Notify you
or tarry stoo
feet, unusual
weakness, bre
this medicati
   In the unl
drug, seek me
reaction incl
breathing.

MEDICATION:
ALPRAZOLAM 0.25 MG TABLET, #00603-2127-21

IMPORTANT:
HOW TO USE THIS INFORMATION: THIS IS A SUMMARY
ABOUT THIS PRODUCT.

COMMON BRAND NAME(S):
Xanax

USES:
Alprazolam is used to treat anxiety and panic disorders. It belong
brain and nerves (central nervous system) to produce a calmi
chemical in the body (GABA).

HOW TO USE:
Take this medication by mouth as directed by your doctor. Dosa
Your dose may be gradually increased until the drug starts work
of side effects.   This medication may cause withdrawal rea
doses. In such cases, withdrawal symptoms (such as seizur
withdrawal reactions, your doctor may reduce your dose gra
benefits, this medication may rarely cause abnormal drug
abused alcohol or drugs in the past. Take this medicatio
medication is used for a long time, it may not work as well.
doctor if your condition persists or worsens.

SIDE EFFECTS:
Drowsiness, dizziness, increased saliva production, or cha
worsen, tell your doctor or pharmacist promptly.   To mini
seated or lying position.   Remember that your doctor has pr
you is greater than the risk of side effects. Many people usi
right away if any of these unlikely but serious side effects oc
slurred speech or difficulty talking, loss of coordination, trou
rare but very serious side effects occur: yellowing eyes or skin,
However, get medical help right away if you notice any symptoms of a serious allergic reaction,
(especially of the face tongue throat), severe dizziness, trouble breathing.   This is not a complete
notice other effects not listed above, contact your doctor or pharmacist.   In the US — Call you
side effects. You may report side effects to FDA at 1-800-FDA-1088.   In Canada - Call your doctor for medical advice about side
effects. You may report side effects to Health Canada at 1-866-234-2345.

PRECAUTIONS:
Before taking alprazolam, tell your doctor or pharmacist if you are allergic to it; or to other benzodiazepines (such as diazepam,
lorazepam); or if you have any other allergies. This product may contain inactive ingredients, which can cause allergic reactions or

LORAZEPAM

(lor a' ze pam)

OTHER NAME : Ativan

WHY is this drug prescribed?
Lorazepam is used to relieve anxiety and insomnia caused by anxiety. It also is used to treat certain side effects of antipsychotic medications.

WHEN should it be used?
For anxiety, lorazepam usually is taken two or three times a day, including a dose at bedtime. For insomnia, it is taken once a day at bedtime. Follow the instructions on your prescription label carefully, an ask your pharmacis
understand. Do not
consulting your do
your doctor, espec
Stopping the drug
symptoms. Your doc

HOW should it be u
Lorazepam comes in
take at each dose.
refilling your pre

What SPECIAL INSTR
Lorazepam can caus
Do not drive a car
drug affects you.
drowsiness caused
not take more of i
longer time than a
the laboratory. Yo
may have blood tes
this medication on
other occasions wh

What should I do I
Do not take a miss
take the next dose

What SIDE EFFECTS
Drowsiness, muscle
dizziness, faintne
contact your docto
trembling, muscle
medication and con

What OTHER PRECAUT
Women who are preg
pregnant, or are b
lorazepam. If you
Before you take th
prescription and r
levodopa, seizure
medication, medica
sedatives, antihis
smoke while taking

Dronabinol (Oral)

Dronabinol (droe-NAB-i-nol) is used to prevent the nausea and vomiting caused by cancer medicines. It is used only when other kinds of medicine for nausea and vomiting do not work. Dronabinol is also used to increase the appetites of patients with AIDS (acquired immunodeficiency syndrome).

Tell your doctor, nurse, and pharmacist if you:
   _ have allergies.
   _ are pregnant or plan to become pregnant.
   _ are breast-feeding
   _ are taking any other medicine, including those you buy yourself such
     as aspirin or cold medicine.
   _ have any other medical problems.

Take this medicine:
   _ exactly the way your doctor told you.

Warning:
   _ If you miss a dose of this medicine, take it as soon as possible.
     However, if it is almost time for your next dose, skip the missed
     dose. Do not double doses.
   _ Do not drink alcohol or take other medicines that make you sleepy.
   _ Do not drive or do dangerous jobs if this medicine makes you dizzy
     or sleepy.
   _ Do not get up fast when you are sitting or lying down. You may faint
     or get dizzy.
   _ If you think you or someone else may have taken an overdose of this
     medicine, get emergency help right away. Some signs of overdose are:
     confusion, changes in mood, hallucinations, mental depression,
     nervousness or anxiety, and fast or pounding heartbeat.
   _ Do not give any of your medicine to others. It may hurt them.
   _ Do not leave this medicine where children can get it.

Tell your doctor right away if you notice any of these possible side effects:
   Less common--Changes in mood; confusion, nervousness, or anxiety; fast
     or pounding heartbeat; hallucinations; mental depression
Some side effects are not serious. However, tell your doctor if these bother you or do not go away:
   More common--Clumsiness or unsteadiness; dizziness; drowsiness;
     trouble in thinking
*** More Information Follows ***

ANTIHISTAMINES - ORAL

USES: This medication provides relief of symptoms of allergic reactions such as rash, hives, watery eyes, runny nose, itchy eyes and sneezing. It may also be used to treat motion sickness, relief of anxiety or tension, or sleeplessness.

HOW TO TAKE THIS MEDICATION: May be taken with food or milk if stomach upset occurs.
   Sustained-release or long acting tablets and capsules must be swallowed whole. Chewing or crushing them will destroy the long action and may increase side effects.
   Shake suspensions well before taking.

SIDE EFFECTS: May cause drowsiness, dizziness, headache, loss of appetite (less likely with cyproheptadine), stomach upset, vision changes, irrit
subside as you
become bothers
   Notify your
pounding, irre
urinating whil

PRECAUTIONS:
as test result
   Change from
dizziness. Use
alertness. Lim
avoid excessiv
   If you have

MEDICATION:
HYDROXYCHLOROQUINE 200 MG TAB, #00378-0373-01

IMPORTANT:
HOW TO USE THIS INFORMATION: THIS IS A SUMMARY AND DOES NOT HAVE ALL POSSIBLE INFORMAT
ABOUT THIS PRODUCT.

COMMON BRAND NAME(S):
Plaquenil

USES:
Hydroxychloroquine is used to prevent or treat malaria infections caused by mosquito bites. It does not work against certain typ malaria (chloroquine-resistant). The United States Center for Disease Control provides updated guidelines and t recommendations for the prevention and treatment of malaria in different parts of the world. Discuss the most recent informa
nalaria occurs.   This medication is also used, usually with other medication
natoid arthritis) when other medications have not worked or cannot be use
- modifying antirheumatic drugs (DMARDs). It can reduce skin problems in l
not known exactly how the drug works.

listed in the approved professional labeling for the drug, but may be prescrib
s condition that is listed in this section only if it has been so prescribed by
lso be used for other types of infections (e.g., Q fever endocarditis).

milk to prevent stomach upset. The dosage and length of treatment are base
In children, dosage is also based on weight. For malaria prevention, take
Mark a calendar to help
weekly while in the area,
t malaria, follow your do
wice daily or as directed.
d your condition has impro
fewest side effects. Use
e, take it at the same time
or, especially if you are taki
ation or treatment too soon
ns. It may take several wee
t prevent malaria in all cas
a different medication. A

effects persist or worsen, n

Dr. Erba

Chemo finished

Check ups + cat scan
    every 3 mo for 2 years
           6 mo for 3 years
           1 yr @ 5 years

    until 7 year mark

if all clean at 7 years - "safe
                            mark"

no remission -
@ 7 years: "LTDFS"

"Long Term Disease Free Survival"

Next:
    Gallium Scan - radioactive picture

    Keep port for a while - still have
        high risk for hospitalization

    Begin radiation in 24 weeks

Start mammograms @ 30 yrs

74

-2-

DR. LICHTER Relapse rate = 30% when Hodgkins is treated w/ chemo
        - typically another treatment ("bone marrow" transplant)
        - good possibility that you're cured
        - if relapse, there is this other treatment
            (50-60% survival rate; overall rate high)
    If radiation: drop relapse rate to 15%
        - if patient fails that, "bone marrow" treatment
          still possible ... but cells more resistant
    Unable to prove that radiation helps ... #s
        end up being around 85%.

    TWO WAYS OF LOOKING AT IT:
        (1) I'm done w/ therapy for now; I'll use
             other therapy if need be
        (2) I'll cut my relapse rate to 15%.
             Brief 4 wks., 5 days a week, few minutes

    Risks: (1) Hodgkins patients increase risk of other
           cancers; hard to say by what percent (small
           but measurable); 10 yrs. out may increase
           risk from 10% to 15-20% for other cancers
         - easily measurable b/c of young population:
           not supposed to have cancer yet

           "Small but acceptable" risk

        (2) W/ diseases like lupus: "suspicion in our literature"
            that they don't respond as well to radiation
            (e.g. breast cancer radiation → scarring, fibrosis)
            (e.g. cervical cancer radiation → no extra effect)
          - once radiation is in, it doesn't come out

BOTTOM LINE: 50% yes, 50% no
        among Hodgkins patients

Q: How much difference does size of tumor make?
   Larger tumor = larger risk
   (massive = greater than 1/3 of chest)

Dr. Lichter: "in general, I recommend this treatmet"
   Q: If 27-yr.-old daughter ... "yes"
Other fine institutions would say "no"

If you decide "yes", Dr. Lichter would want
to consult w/ colleagues about your special
case (Lupus).

So... you decide independent of Lupus; if "yes,"
then he'll do research

Q: what are 2ndary cancers?
   breast, lung, thyroid, colon
   ‾‾‾‾‾ ‾‾‾‾
     most common

Q: relapse of Hodgkins: better or worse than 2ndary cancers?
   breast cancer treatable, but some deaths
   lung cancer serious

More chemo. options: higher dose, cytoxin, mop(?), ...

► Ask Dr. Irbe (?) his opinion

Q: when to begin? could start after Jan. 5
Q: Risk to reproductive organs? NO
Q: Side effects? fatigue swallowing nausea

For Dad, when he gets back: you have a healthy baby girl!

15-Jan-2002

Patient Type: A
Location:

LIEBERMAN, JESSICA
DOB: 7-Jun-1971 Sex: F
70315700

MRN: 2047461

Hx: PT HAS HODGKIN'S DZ
    ASSESS DZ PROGRESSION
    201.91

1/8/02 CT OF THE CHEST, ABDOMEN AND PELVIS

HISTORY: Hodgkin's disease. Evaluate status of disease.

COMPARISON: None

PROCEDURE: IV and oral contrast. Apex of lungs to bottom of pelvis.

FINDINGS

CHEST: Calcified 3 mm. left lower lobe pulmonary nodule (image 30).
Non-calcified 2 mm. left upper lobe pulmonary nodule (image 10).
Slight prominence to tissue in the region of the thymus. This may be
residual thymus or treated tumor. This measures 1.1 x 1.7 cm. (image
12). No middle mediastinal or hilar adenopathy. Heart and
pericardium normal. Axilla and supraclavicular fossa normal.

ABDOMEN: Liver, kidneys, adrenal glands, spleen, pancreas,
gallbladder normal. No upper abdominal lymphadenopathy.

PELVIS: No pelvic lymphadenopathy. Uterus, bladder, ovaries and
pelvic bowel within normal limits.

IMPRESSION:

Mild prominence to soft tissue in the anterior mediastinum. This may
represent treated lymphoma, or rebound hyperplasia of the thymus.
I have no prior to compare to to see if this is growing, shrinking or
unchanged.

77

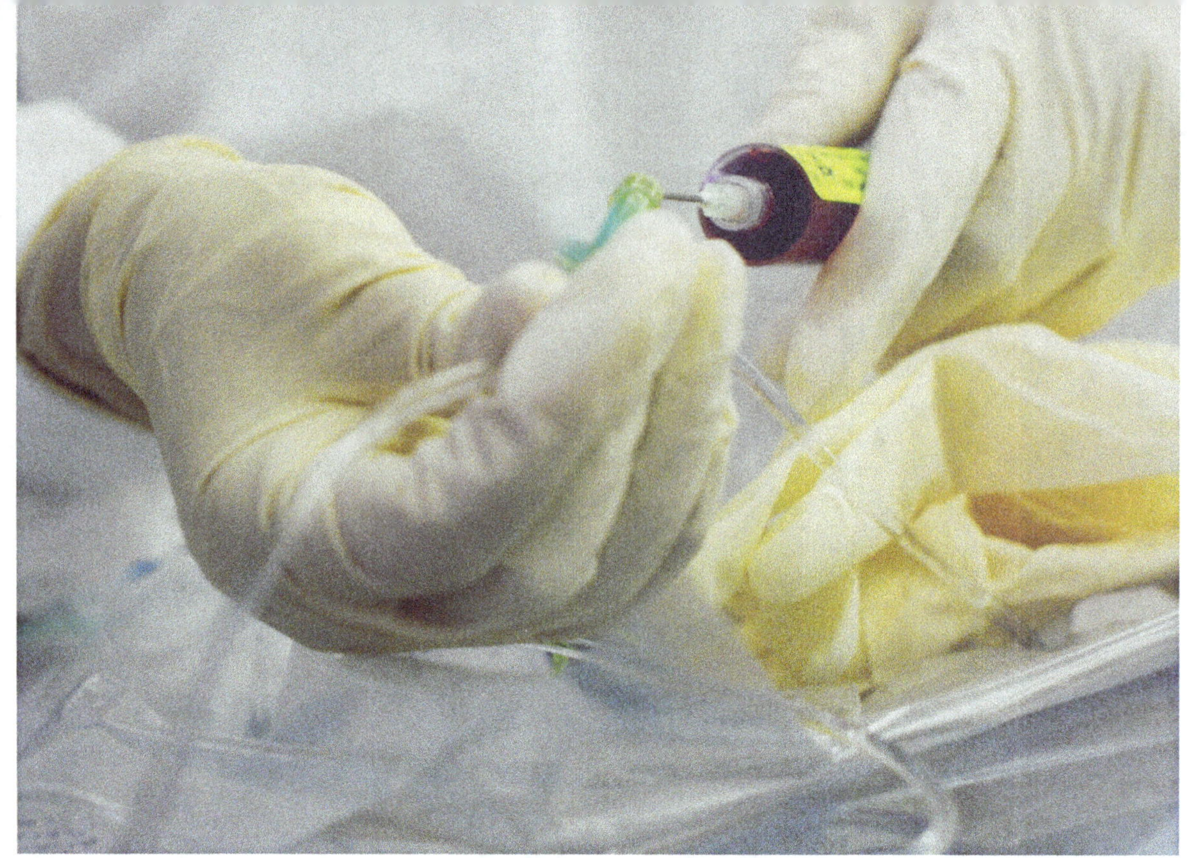

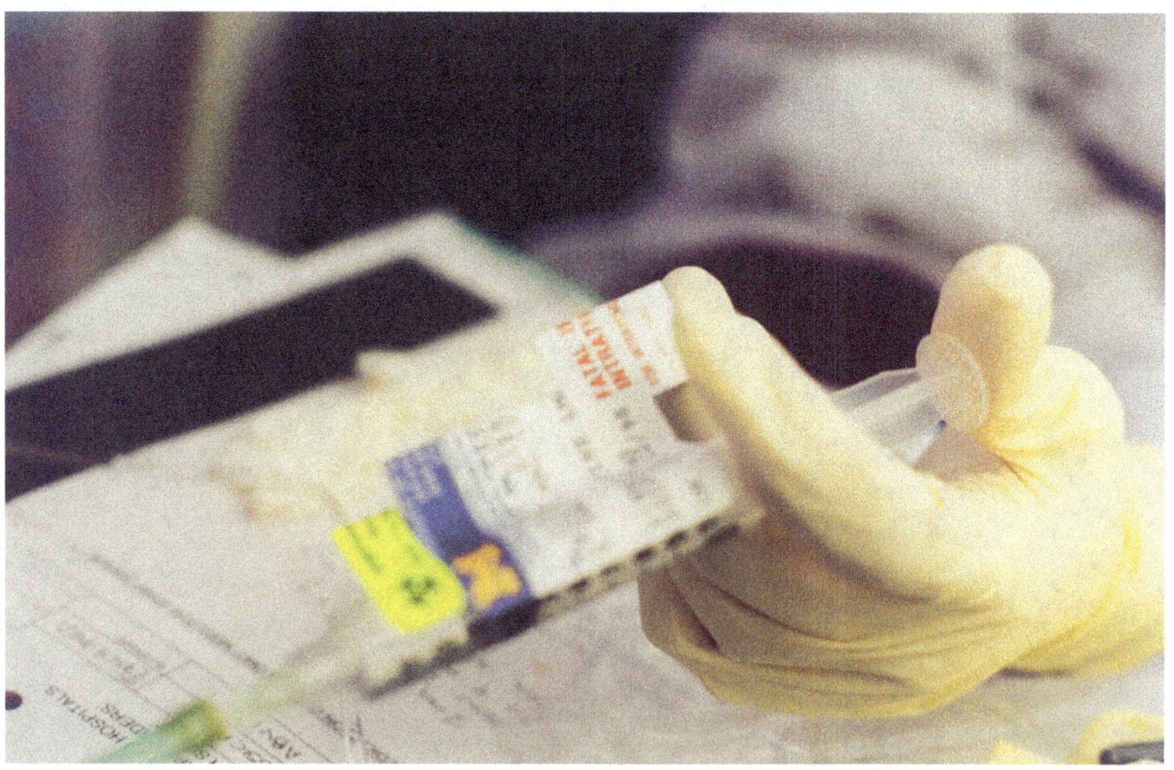

FATAL
INTR

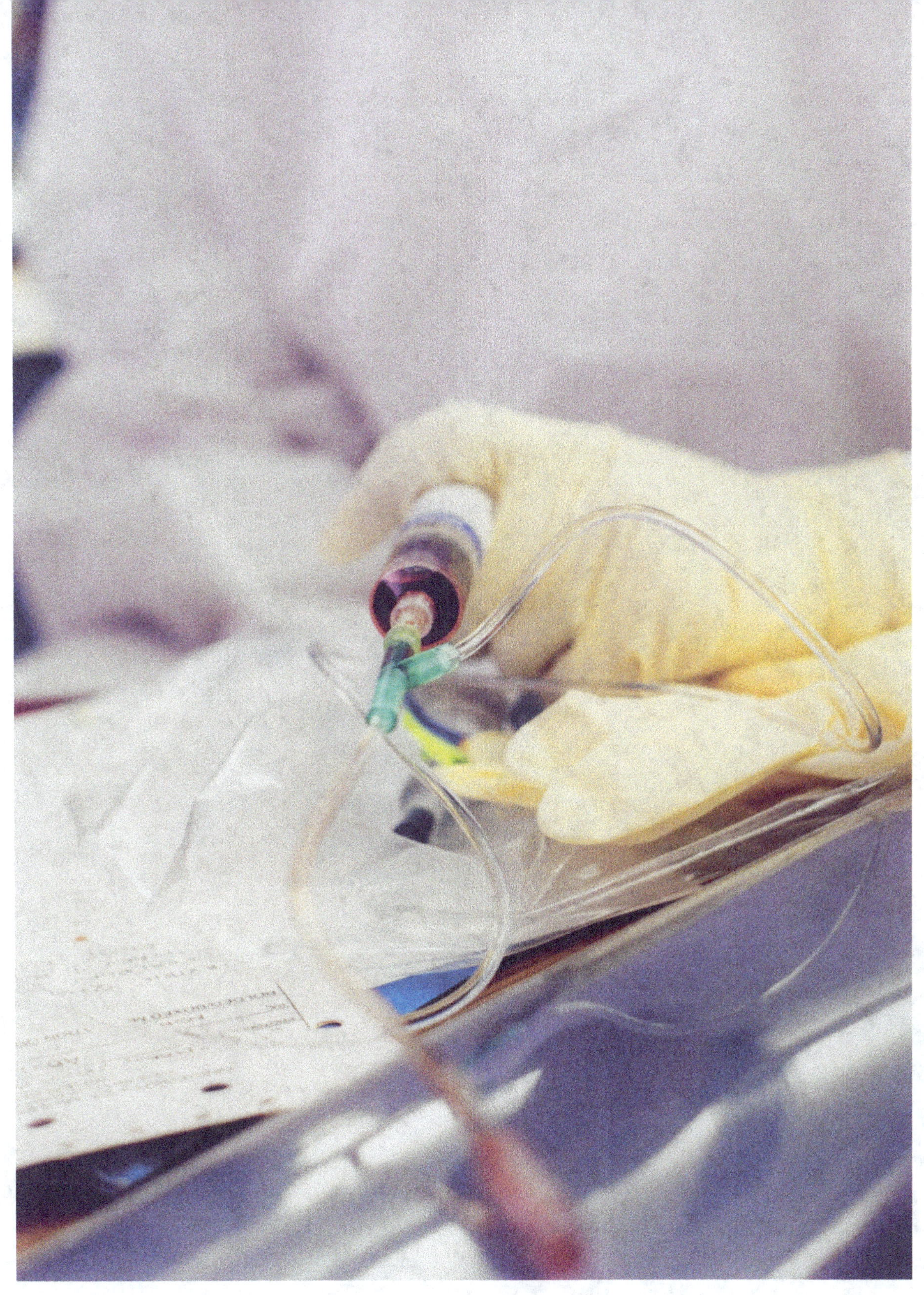

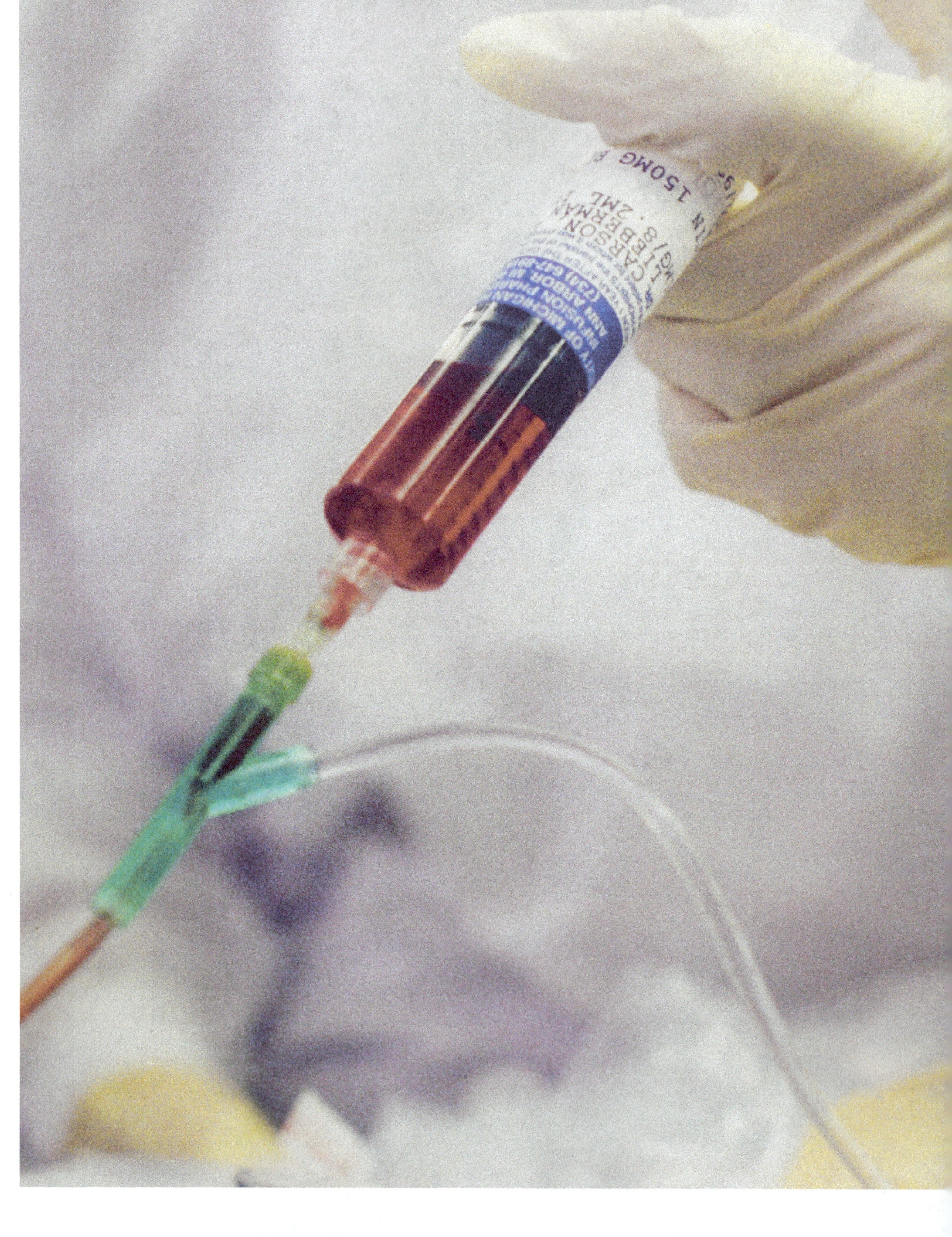

Nearing the End / Icons

Sleep feels like waiting to me now. I, who could sleep in the movie theater, the car, on the telephone, in front of the TV, even in loud rooms full of people talking and music blasting. I cannot sleep anymore. It is no longer the anxiety. And I have no specific aches or pains that make positioning impossible. It's as if I have simply finished sleeping. For now, for tonight, for the term of this illness.

I always try to force it, lying in bed for an hour or so, my mind racing with the most banal details of class announcements, prescriptions to be refilled, errands undone. My thoughts inevitably turn to teaching—that saving grace that provides not simply distraction, but also a calm determination and sense of accomplishment. So, while I fight the wakefulness as long as I can, it is this more disturbing invasion of my peace that forces me out of bed: better to perform the now soothing tasks that build up when teaching than to lie by uselessly as my mind unravels their serenity and categorizes their atomized parts into daunting lists of "things to do."

I am just so tired. Neither sleep nor wakefulness holds much meaning anymore. They are like icons emptied of their context. Powerful placeholders for sets of meaning no longer close at hand.

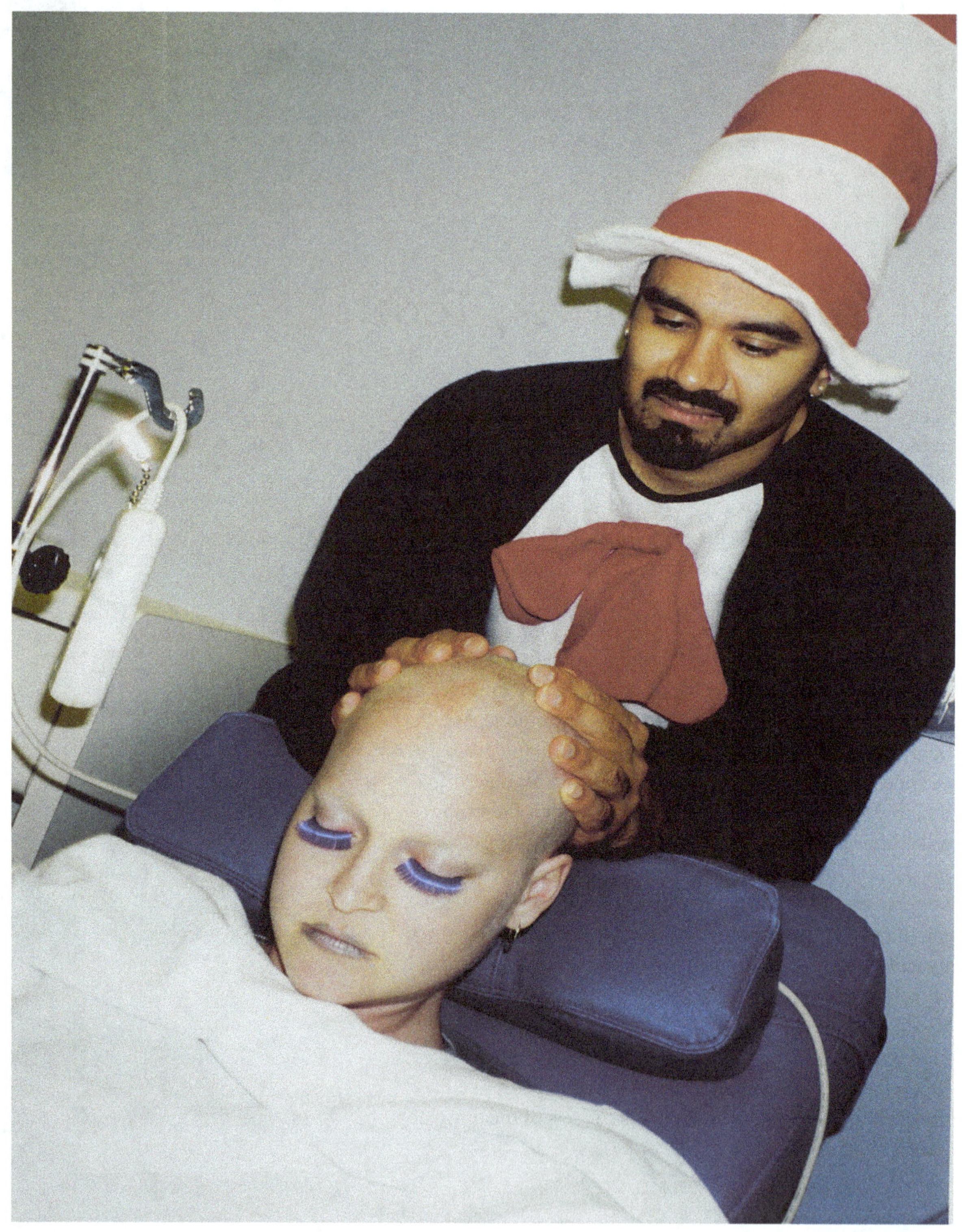

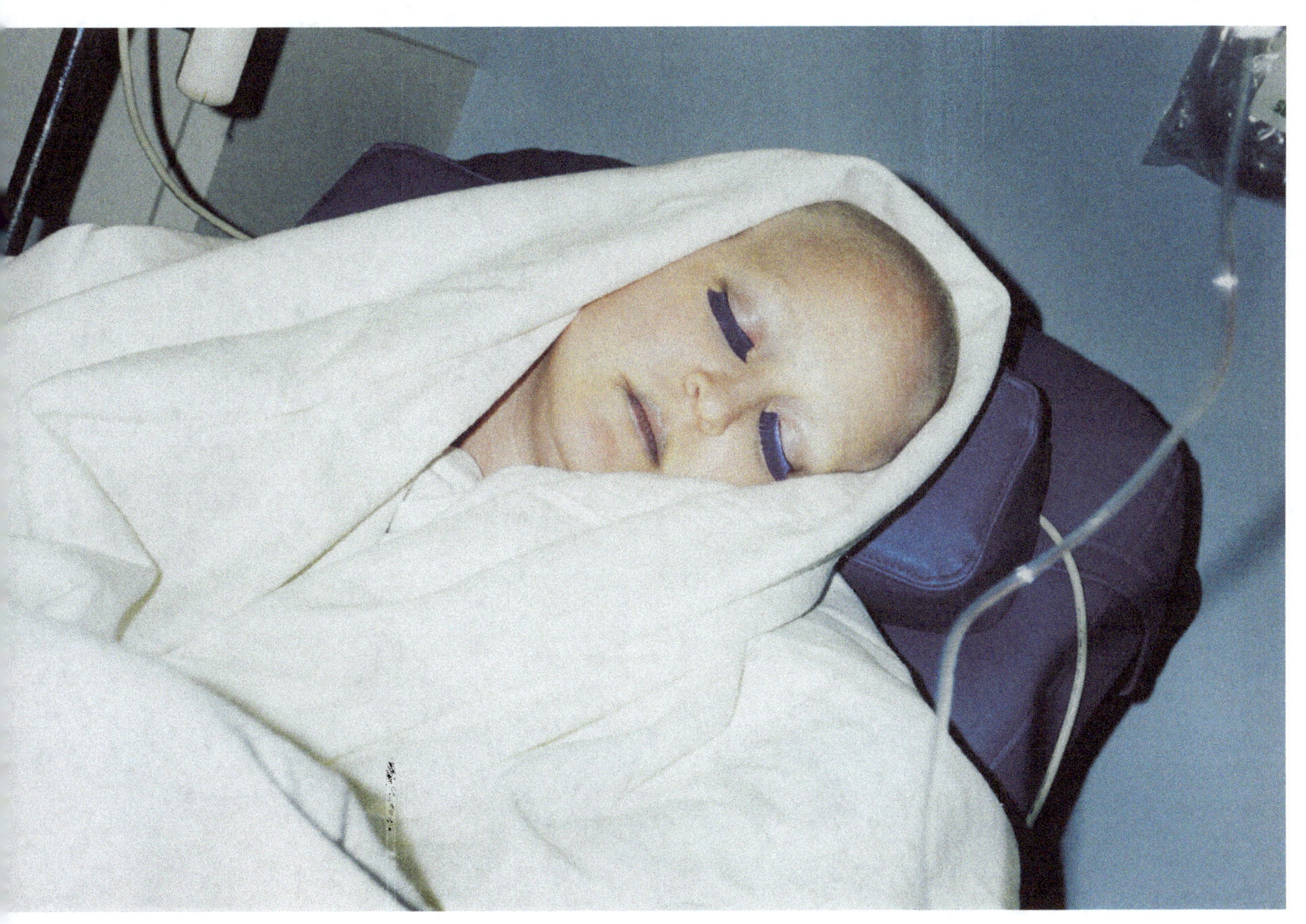

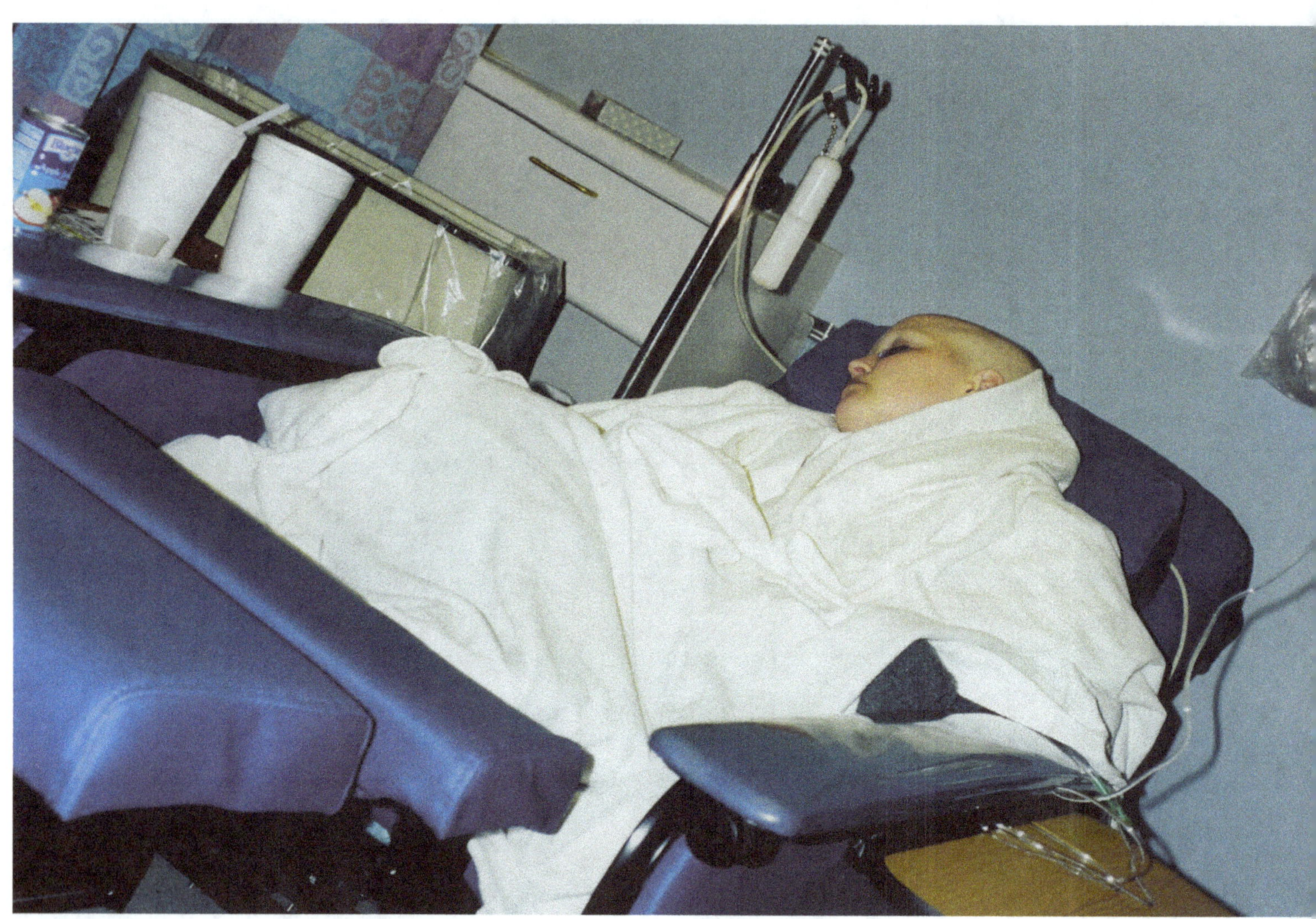

86

Radiation

I DID NOT TAKE A SINGLE PICTURE of my time in radiation—the only images I have are afterthoughts. A Polaroid was taken by one of my radiology technicians as a visual aid for his calculations: it marked his target and allowed him a sense of its location on the plane of my chest. The next day, those marks were tattooed permanently onto my flesh and the photo was thrown away. I took it out of the trash bin.

The second image I have is a memento of sorts. When I finished radiation, the techs asked if I wanted to keep my "bed." They felt bad that they had confiscated my camera so many times, and this was something they could give to me. I took it. It was about four and a half feet tall and three feet wide and filled with a hardened, diarrhea-yellow foam that had grown around my naked body as two techs mixed unknown liquids to produce a rather impressive chemical reaction. But it was large and very bulky, and I had to ask someone to carry it home for me. With nowhere to store such a thing in a shared studio apartment, I put it out with the trash. When I returned home from a CT scan, I found it lying flat on the sidewalk, a sarcophagus radiating in the sun.

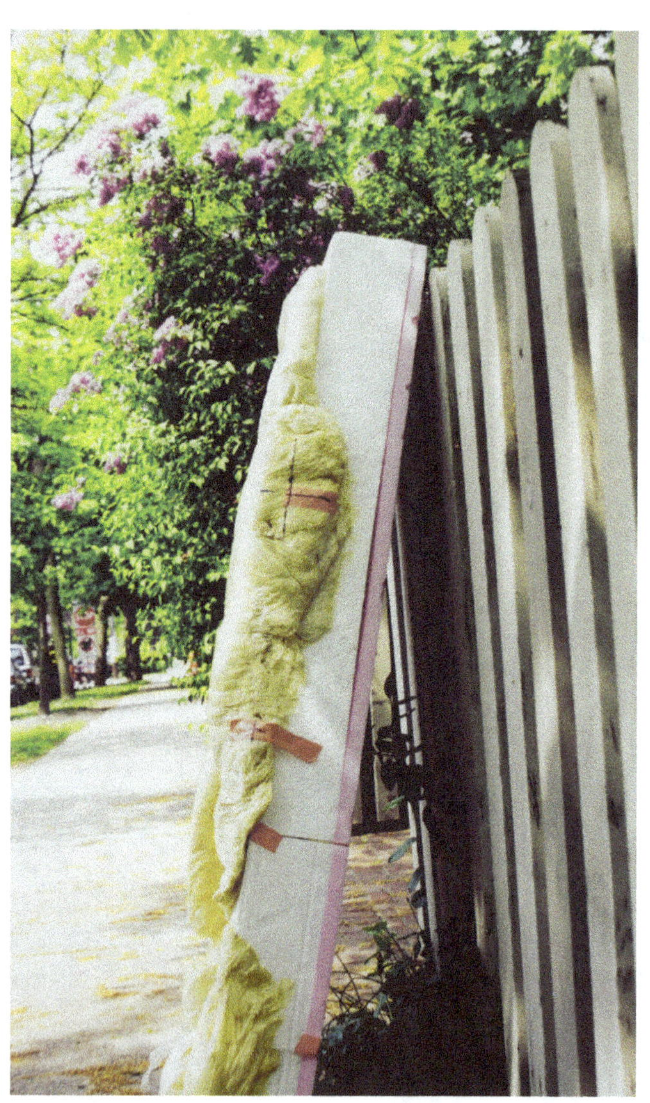

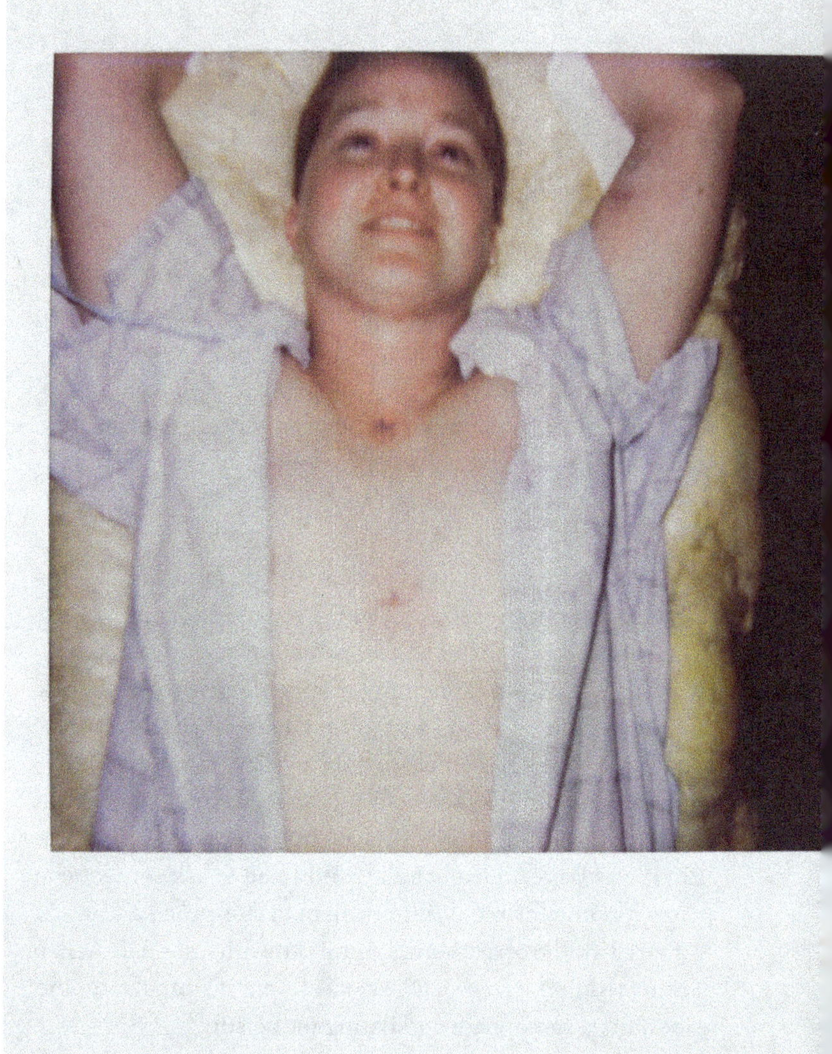

90

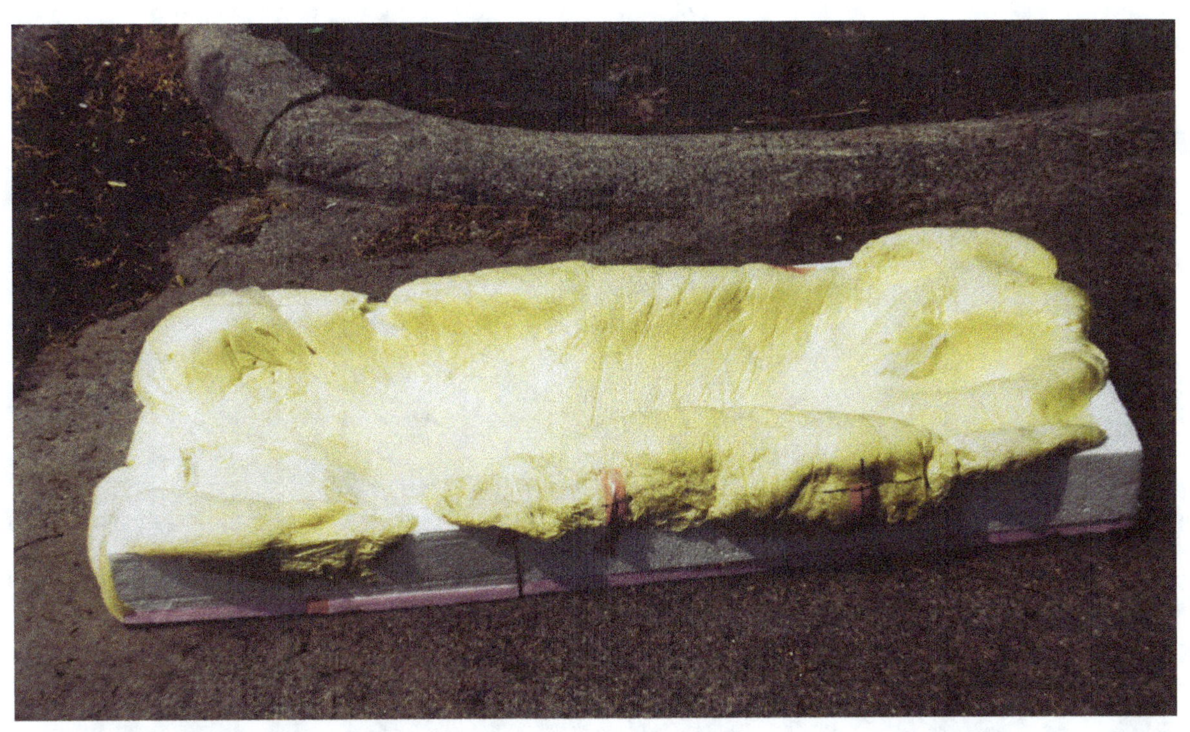

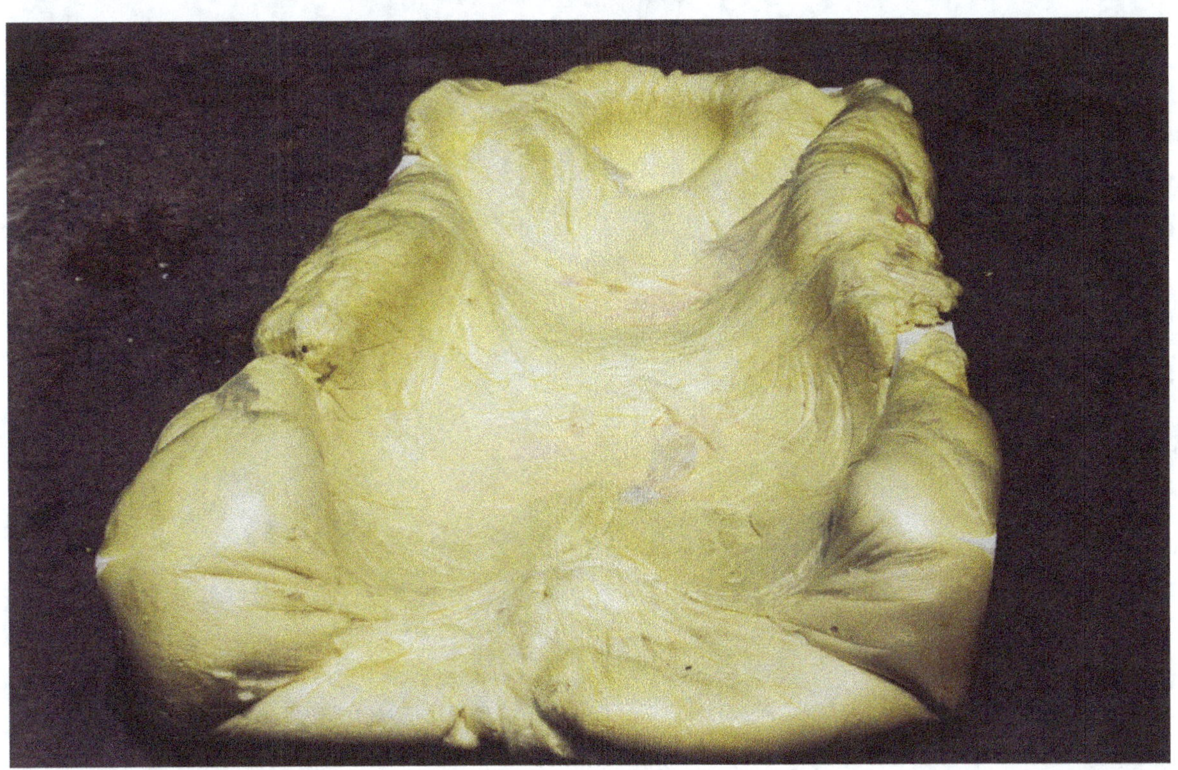

CONVERSATION

THERE WERE SIX OF US: two old women, one old man,
one middle-aged woman, one middle-aged man, and me.
There were five of them: two husbands, one wife, one
brother, and one boyfriend. By the third day of sitting together in radiation's cramped waiting room, we had begun
to talk. Just a couple of us at first, then a few more. One of
the old women never did speak, not once in the four weeks
we spent together. Nor did she ever arrive accompanied by
a loved one. During a February blizzard, as my boyfriend
half-carried me to our car, I saw her waiting in the parking
lot. A hired van was lowering a ramp to let her in. I never
learned her name.

It took me three months to gain the right combination
of confidence, defiance, ingenuity, and audacity to begin
making images in the chemotherapy wing of the Cancer
Center. I never gained any of that in radiology. I would like
to have made portraits of Ruth, the middle-aged woman,
and her husband, John. Of Jim and Mary, the elderly couple.
Though I do not want to ever see a photograph of Mickey,
the middle-aged man who died twice in our waiting room.
If it were not for him, I might have asked Ruth about a
portrait, though she would never have understood. Jim and
Mary would have posed without a thought. But Mickey was
always there.

Mickey was the "worst off" of our group. He was too far gone and the treatment was irrelevant. But, he explained, he needed something to do. He had not slept in six weeks, since his diagnosis. When he left his construction job early one day to see a doctor about back pain, he was given a diagnosis of metastasized lung cancer and three weeks to live. He stayed awake for those three weeks, feeding himself off of anxiety and morphine. Now he had a morphine pump in his spine, a full body cast from knee to top of head that served as an exoskeleton in lieu of his own cancer-riddled bones, and a bleary-eyed stare that revealed an overdose of drugs, sleeplessness, and rumination. The first time Ruth and I struck up conversation, Mickey flashed to life and joined us. Each day when I arrived, his brother-in-law, a large Native American man in work clothes who drove in two and a half hours each day to sit with the shrinking and pasty-white Mickey, would nudge him into awareness. Mickey would then tell me about his constipation, diarrhea, waking wet dreams, and pain. I would nod my head in sympathy until he was called in for his placebo treatment. He always left just as Jim was coming in from the changing room. Jim must have been in his seventies, but he had great legs—muscular legs that sprawled out awkwardly in the absurd hospital gown that he wore for treatment. He looked lovely but exposed. Mary would smile as she watched me observe her husband and then say something heartfelt about Mickey.

It was Ruth who became my friend. She was feisty and bitter, sarcastic and angry. Infuriated by her condition, she blamed all doctors for her lung cancer and whined for cigarettes. She was hot-tempered and dismissive of Mickey because she was dying too, and she knew it. Her husband John did not. My partner and John would commiserate affably about the workload cancer had left them: cooking, cleaning, massaging, and near-daily trips to the pharmacy for prescriptions. Ruth would tell me about her appointments and the ineptitude of her doctors. Every day she decided, "Enough is enough . . . I'm lookin' into hospice." She was supposed to finish radiation two days after I met her. She

94

was supposed to begin chemotherapy. But she showed up
the following Monday in her silly radiation gown. Over the
weekend she had begun to drool and within hours had lost
her ability to speak clearly. By Monday morning, the right
side of her face was paralyzed and sagging, and her chemo
doctors sent her back to radiation. Her lung cancer had
metastasized and chemotherapy could not treat the tumors
in her brain. For the duration of our friendship, Ruth spat
saliva in my face while trying not to become incomprehen-
sible when her anger got her too excited to speak slowly.
Two weeks into our friendship, she came in talking about
her meeting with the hospice people. She blew me a kiss as
I went in for my treatment and I never saw her again.

That Wednesday Mickey died. This time, for good.

I had a week and a half of radiation left. I walked into the
waiting room each morning with my heavy winter coat
hood pulled over my head and waited for my partner to get
his coffee. When he came in, I lay down on an empty couch,
hospital gown tucked between my legs, and slept with my
head in his lap until my techs called me in. New patients
filled the vacated time slots and joined us in the tiny room.
I don't remember any of them.

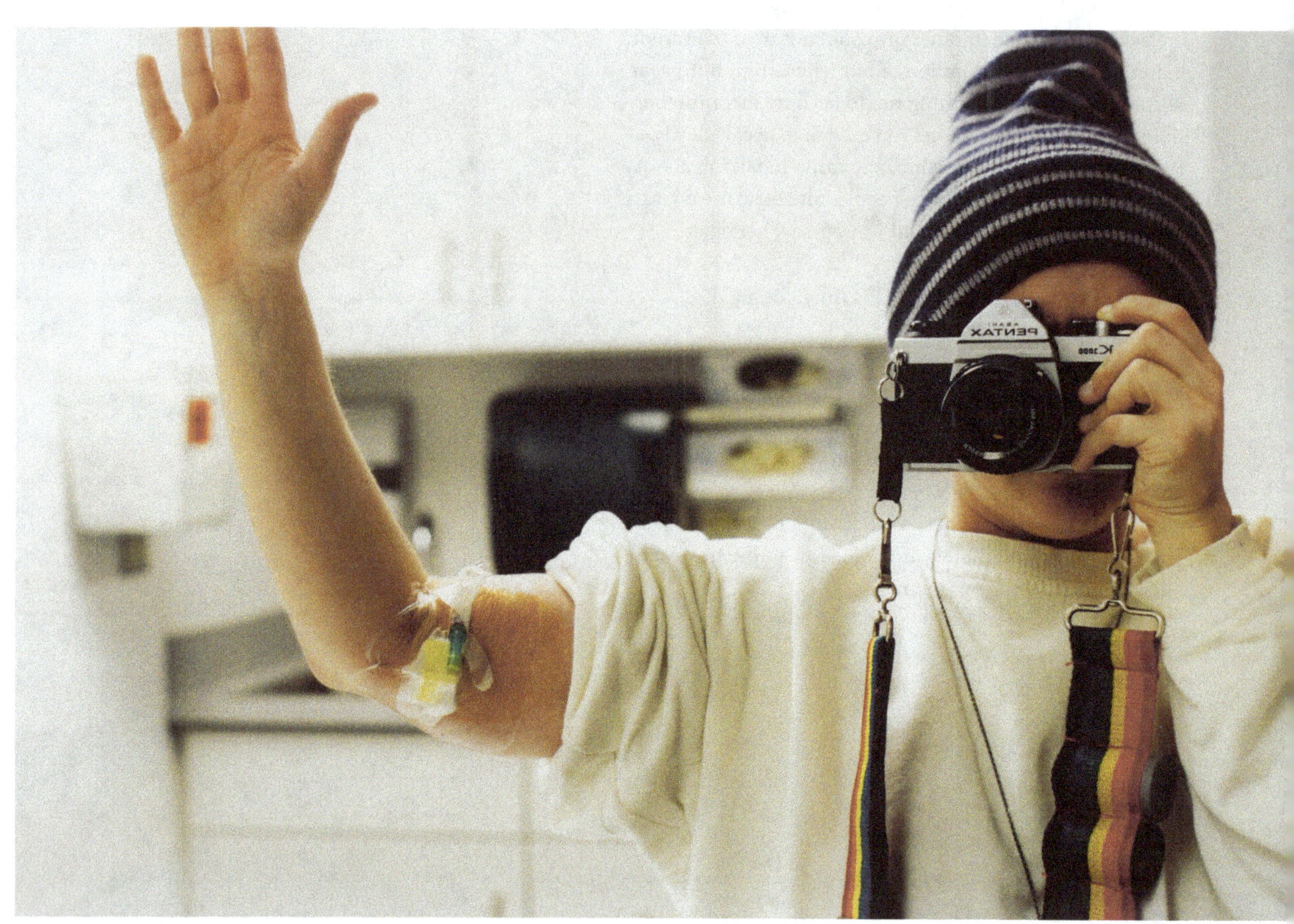

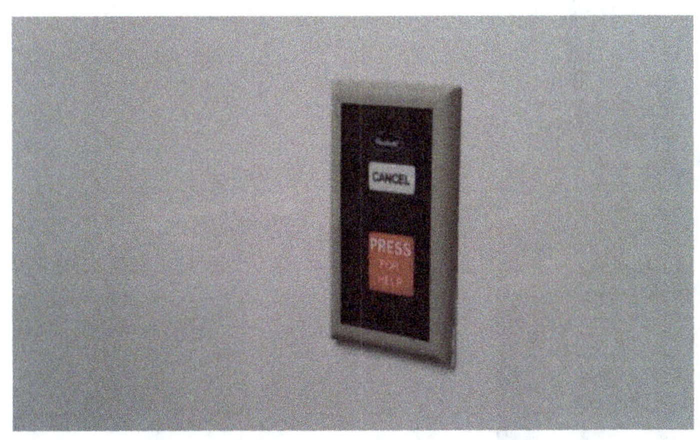

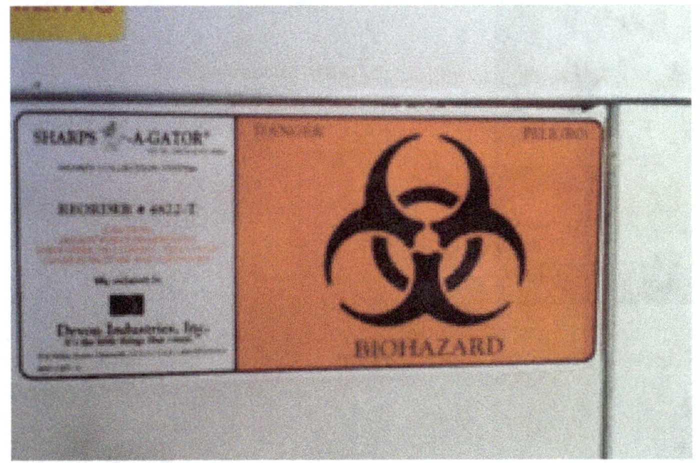

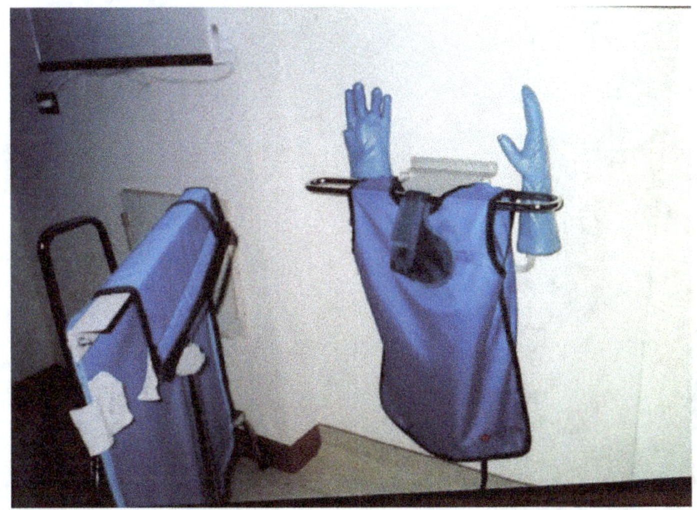

97

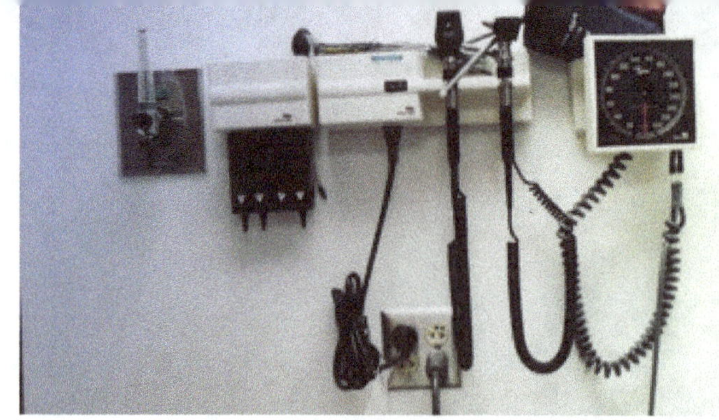
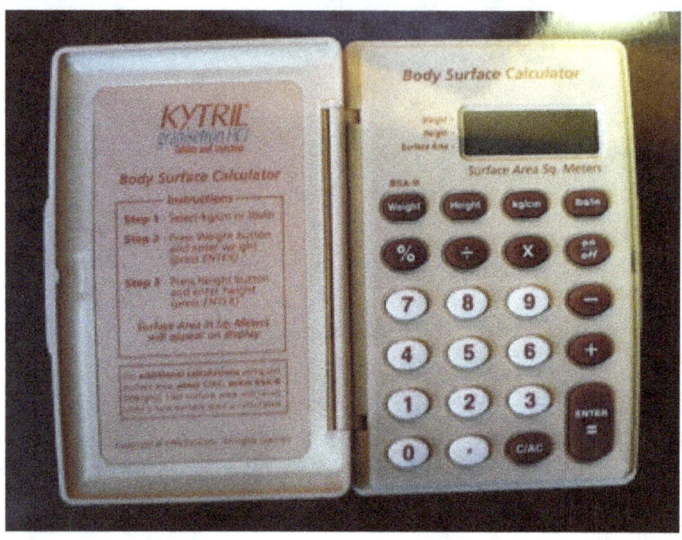

KYTRIL
Body Surface Calculator
Instructions
Body Surface Calculator
Surface Area Sq. Meters

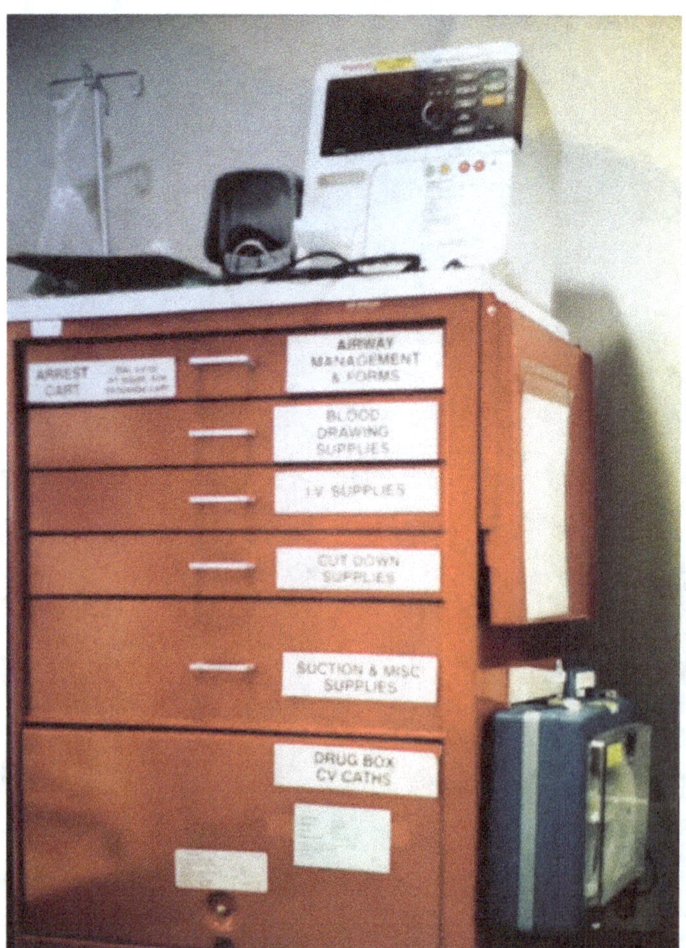

ARREST CART
AIRWAY MANAGEMENT & FORMS
BLOOD DRAWING SUPPLIES
IV SUPPLIES
CUT DOWN SUPPLIES
SUCTION & MISC SUPPLIES
DRUG BOX CV CATHS

Dear Jeff—

How wonderful you are! I have just spent two hours whirl-
ing around my apartment, dancing and singing and pant-
ing and gasping to the CD you sent. Now I am out of breath
and nauseated, but completely happy. I spent the morning
grading student papers while feeling sick and annoyed,
pissed off that none of my doctors will tell me my test
results and it's been five full days of waiting. Then "One
Way Street" came on and I prepared to sing my lungs out
but started sobbing instead, really sobbing, and not for any
reasons that make sense, but for strange reasons, illusive,
allusive, elusive. Though the song meant something different to your daughter when she wrote it, what I hear now is
her voice, the stirring voice of a survivor, entreating, "Tell
me, tell me what it is that you see through me, through the
choice I made," just as I am questioning my decision to
continue treatment and wanting to pull the plug on radiation. But Emily's voice coaxes, "Don't look back . . . hold
your course, the road is long and there are cracks . . . and if
you're tempted, remember what I said, I am here."

How vividly I remember listening to the song and singing with all my heart while driving through Yellowstone
National Park only a year and a half ago. I felt so healthy,
alive, strong, and immune as I thought about Emily and her
Hodgkin's diagnosis. She was so sick and I was so far away
from her experience. I would listen to "Inside Out" and
think of chemotherapy and baldness and hospitals and cry
for Emily's experience: "Words travel through air, spoken
in whispers, so carefully . . . still, they weigh so much, that

I'm awakened by the sound, of a harmony—where nothing seems in tune . . . Inside out, can't figure out, how to
say what's true and console you . . . make you see what's
really me." I would think of her beauty, and her voice and
her music and I would cry for her. And now I am crying to
the same song but from such a different place. Now she is
healthy and recording albums and I am dying . . . or recovering. Now she is a person I know in ways so many people
will never know and her songs overwhelm me in whole new
ways. "Strange as it seems, there lies a gift in this, an ability,
to see hear taste and touch, without a single sense to call
upon." She is becoming visible to me now in whole new
ways and, in her words, I understand myself as someone
who can be seen and heard. I am acutely aware of the difference in myself listening now—a self so other than the one
who sang along before—and am so grateful to you and your
family for the continued letters, gifts, and well wishes . . .
but also for having lived this before me.

Visibly,
Jess

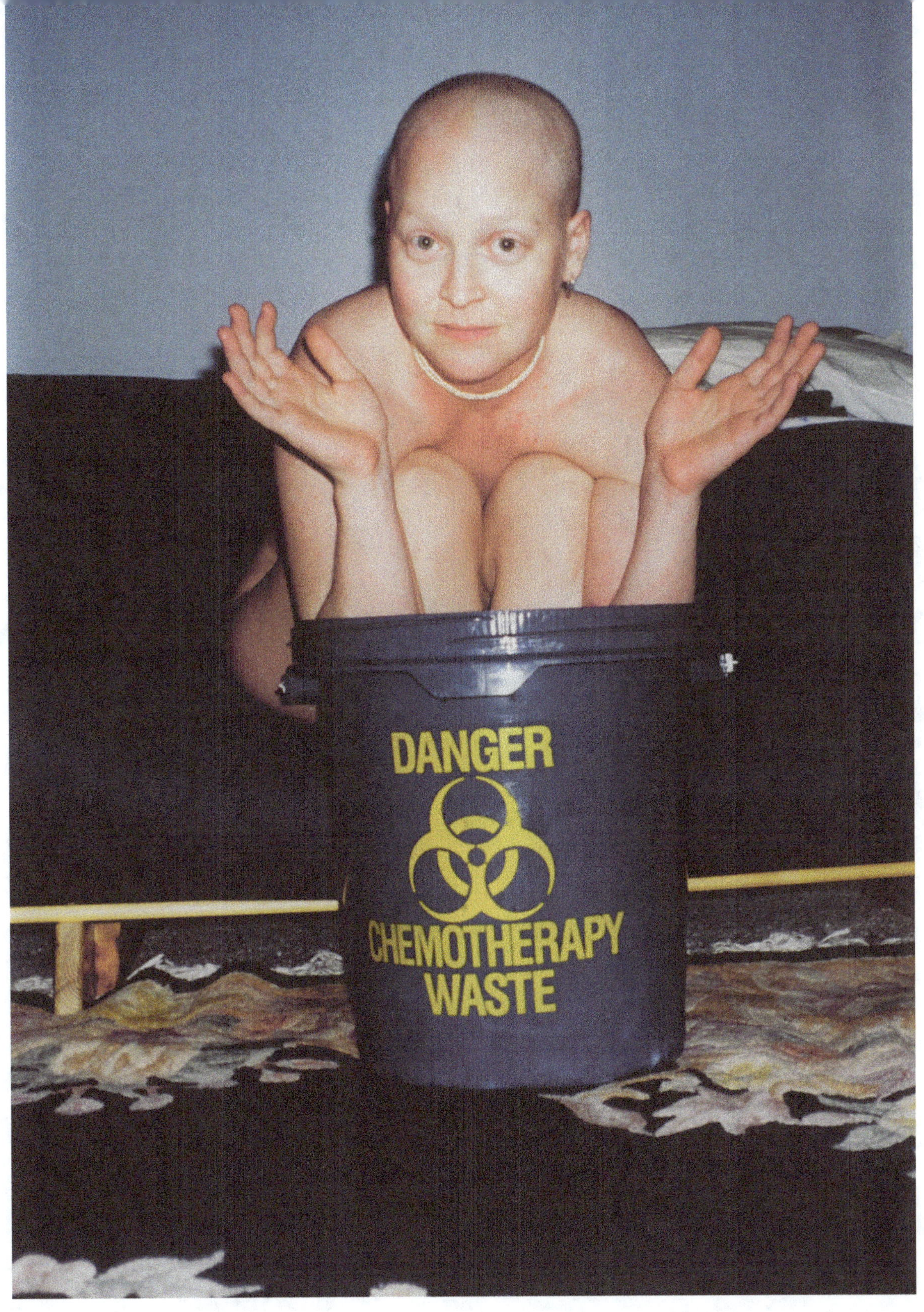

DANGER
CHEMOTHERAPY
WASTE

Afterword

IN LATE NOVEMBER 2012, I am finalizing the syllabus for a winter-term session of my undergraduate seminar, The Art of Dying. I am carefully plotting an agenda for the next three months, scheduling film viewings and student presentations to coincide with days when I will be recovering from surgery and more fit to listen than to lecture. While looking for spaces to squeeze in the newest work by artists this year and substituting the newest critical discussions for some of the less impactful readings of the past, I scan the course outline of dead and dying artists as if it is an autonomous, amalgamated body, breathing and wheezing and calling out to me in need of a couple Advil and a routine visit to a primary care physician.

It is a successful class. In its fifth year, it is perpetually over-enrolled and often carries a wait list. The usual suspects—photography, design, film and museum studies majors; minors in art history and in women's and gender studies—are joined by students from across our university, engineers, business majors, game designers, who take an interest in the visual and image-based aspects of their fields. Most of all, they all come ready to talk about death.

My students find that taboos around discussions of death, dying, illness, pain, and disability are prevalent in all of their disciplines and almost every area of their experience. Even my biomedical photographers, who are carefully trained to

shoot in morgues and surgical theaters, report a sustained
denial of questions of living and dying implicit in the very
professional character of their working protocols. Throughout the term, one student will inevitably speak self-deprecat-
ingly about her morbid fascinations; another will mention
his recent experience with serious illness; someone will
relate the tragic events surrounding the suicide of a parent
or friend. Nearly all the members of our class will, at some
point, question the silence and discomfort surrounding
these topics in their families, their social circles, in cultural
practices of mourning and healing. As students grow more
accustomed to the discourse, new silences and erasures
occur to them. They are sometimes frustrated, sometimes
sympathetic, and often deeply empathetic regarding our
shared discomfort with bringing critique to the unspoken
and sad.

Persistent philosophical, psychological, narrative, and
semiotic themes—time, fear, hope, control, enlightenment,
anger, friendship, politics of change, invisibility, objectification—join evolving tropes and genres—ars moriendi,
momento mori, vanitas, danse macabre, "cult" circulation,
"deep" or "dark web" undergrounds—as we explore the
artistic production of individuals who are facing death.
The materials are difficult, the readings complex, the
images disturbing, unsettling, and discomforting.
The ideas are provocative and do not, to quote a student,
"clear the system easily." Rigorously intellectual theory
sometimes jars with highly emotional content. Sometimes
we leave class exhausted, weary. Other times we are ener-
gized, focused, inspired. Most of the time, students simply
don't leave class. We tend to gather afterwards, continue to
unpack the material, discuss other artists, or sometimes
simply unwind.

I created the course with and for my students who were
looking for something they could not find in the curricu-
lum. In 2002 I had developed a seminar I called Traumatic
Images. Students responded powerfully, and while I made
the course a permanent offering, they circulated a petition

asking for Traumatic Images 2. Parsing their feedback from those first few years, I realized that the scholarship and materials most readily available to them centered on the representation of others. Photographic theory, critique of visual cultures, trauma theory, discussions of photojournalism, documentary, and biomedical work, psychoanalytic and feminist and Marxist critique—all were primarily focused on, and best targeted to, a world of witness in which my students and I were posited as viewers, voyeurs, consumers, re-circulators. At the same time, our own lived experience was becoming increasingly "i-reported." Social media and digital technology were mingling with our own narcissistic politics to co-constitute a new manifestation of performing ourselves, specifically, in images by our own hand.

By focusing our lens on visual autopathography, we forge for ourselves a key vantage point from which to study contemporary visual culture, image circulation, and the politics, poetics, and taboos of representation. One can trace the idea of autopathography quite simply from medical textbooks of the mid-nineteenth century, to Freud's popularization of case studies, and on to Oliver Sacks. Arthur W. Frank, G. Thomas Courser, Mark Lawson, Anne Hunsaker Hawkins, Jeffrey K. Aronson, and Rachel Hall-Clifford anchor a very small constellation of scholars who focus their different disciplinary approaches on personal narratives of illness. Notably, however, none of them focuses on visual representation. In constructing The Art of Dying, I find limited content and critique in the realms of pathography, even more limited sources in autopathography, and only a few, mostly buried, handfuls of visual autopathography—a scarcity that may well reflect their transient recognition, intense effect and affect, and the complex conditions of their production. To talk about the taboo complexities of illness and dying is not the norm. To write your own experience and share it publicly is unusual. To share that experience visually, to reveal in and through art, appears to be singular. My students thrive when contemplating this difference. It speaks to their contentious relationship with the images they make, encounter, and interrogate.

A discussion of two of the best-known artists of these visual acts of self-representation, Hannah Wilke and Jo Spence, highlights a potent aspect of visual autopathography's unique politics and dangers. Wilke and Spence spent their photographic careers depicting their own often-naked bodies while navigating the critical landmines of objectification, from Jacques Lacan's traumatic "gaze" to Laura Mulvey's "male gaze." When illness began to change their bodies, each photographer continued to train her lens on her self and her vulnerable form. The double objectification of the gaze became multiplied, adding the concerns of Michel Foucault's "medical gaze" and even E. Ann Kaplan's "imperial gaze" to the strange otherness of their diseased bodies. Each woman's subversive body—obstinately refusing to conform to the standards of conventional femininity, expectations of youthful health and beauty, fears about the loss of control equated with dying—calls out to the viewer as witness. Affective reception is shaped by careful, feminist performances that problematize stereotypical expectations of privacy, class, female bodies, illness, and disease. These images capture the subject of simultaneous life and death (dying as living and living while dying) while reflecting a history of theoretical discourse—from Roland Barthes to Susan Sontag to Ulrich Baer—about photography's uncanny disruption of linear time, ghosting of the present, and representation as death. Wilke and Spence present their suffering and represent their selves without restoration or resolution. They proffer the contradictions of subjectivity, of illness embodied, as a continuous aspect of life—death simultaneous with and constitutive of living.

Issues of witness, of an ethical viewer spurred to action, suggest a hope that visual reception will result not in closure but in the promotion of discourse. In 2013, visual culture scholarship is actively calling for ethical politics in an image-world of disease, war, terror, and torture. Jill Bennett argues for "empathic vision," a practice of visual arts that is "generative rather than representational" (Bennett 2005, 153). She describes how the "affective" operation of the visual process can be political and "shift perception and thereby engender new ways of thinking" (152). In order to conduct "politics through an imagery of affectively charged space" (153), Bennett suggests, contemporary art would do well to engage trauma not as something to communicate to an audience, but as something to "transact." The experience transcribed by an image should excite neither identification nor sympathy in the viewer, but rather "affective responses . . . [that] emerge from a direct engagement with sensation as it is registered in the work" (7).

Lisa Saltzman and Eric Rosenberg also call upon the centrality of visual economies to an understanding of trauma and argue that a "space of trauma is that very domain that exists between the visual and the verbal . . . that trauma itself might emerge from the attempt to navigate that space" (Saltzman and Rosenberg 2006, xii). Charting a history of the relationship between trauma and the visual field, they gather together the work of scholars in search of "the possibility of producing a site of ethical encounter, of conversation, of communication across cultural and traumatic difference" (xvi). Judith Butler uses Emmanuel Levinas's concept of the "face" in search of an ethics of nonviolence and a recognition of the precariousness of life. In the visual encounter with the imaged face of another, she sees not only a site of aggression, but also the potential of ethical struggle and an "instigation to a sensate democracy" (Butler 2004, 151). Martha Rosler and Carol Squiers bring this call for social change to the politics of the body and illness, arguing that pictures should always be combined with social and historical context, advocacy, and analysis (Rosler 2004, 240; Squiers 2005, 17).

Perhaps the most promising potential for politics in the precariousness of life, exemplified by illness and manifest in visual autopathography, is depicted by Eric Cazdyn when he describes our current state of living as the "new chronic." Starting with the medical discourse of illness, he shifts the time frame to better reflect what he sees as our contemporary reality of extending the present into the future: "chronic" instead of "terminal" and "management" instead of "cure." Coping with his own diagnosis of chronic cancer, Cazdyn believes that a re-conception of the relationship between life and death "shakes up the possibility for an active political resistance. . . . The already dead already inhabits revolution—that is, they inhabit a revolutionary consciousness informed by a certain way of living in time and space, and in relation to an unknown and unrealized future" (Cazdyn 2012, 9). This is the discursive terrain in which a study of visual autopathography can now intervene. In visual and verbal provocations, a project such as *Becoming Visible* transacts a traumatic encounter with the unchecked growth and entropic time of cancer, institutional spaces of medicine and bureaucracy, and the power of generative affect in deploying images for empathic witness.

* * *

When I finished my cancer therapy; when chemotherapy and radiation were exhausted; when my images and scans convinced my doctors that it was time for me to switch my primary care to rheumatologists, ophthalmologists, and oral surgeons who would follow my autoimmune disease and permanent side effects while reassigning my hematologists, radiologists, and oncologists to follow-up care duties; when this long moment of my life was over, the surgeons removed my port. During my first chemo treatment, we quickly discovered that my veins would not tolerate the toxic medications. So a surgeon implanted a portacath, or subcutaneous port, into my arm. About the size of a large gumball, the port was placed under my skin and connected to a long, plastic tubing catheter that tunneled through my arm and into a large vein that empties into my heart. The port served as a reception site for the needle that would carry the chemo and other medications and fluids into my heart as well as remove blood for tests. My port spent a year in my body and weathered infection, clots, and blocked lines as my body reacted against and eventually incorporated it. My port spared me time and pain. But it also cost me time and pain. It was a fraught relationship.

When I met with the surgeon prior to its removal, I insisted
that I be allowed to keep the port. As I had come to expect
by this point, he refused to give it to me, citing hospital
protocols, sanitation, potential litigation, etc. After some
negotiation, he agreed that I would be allowed to "see" it
before it was properly disposed of. When a resident brought
it to me later, she told me to return it to a recovery nurse
when I was through. She placed a surgical cloth on my
bedside table. It contained a golf-ball-sized lump of flesh. I
could see a glimpse of the metal port. But it was completely
grown over in the scar tissue and flesh that my body had
adaptively encased it with. I wrapped it back up and placed
it in my post-op aftercare kit.

That evening, back in my apartment, I began removing the
human tissue with manicure scissors. It was remarkably
difficult. The tissue was startlingly tough and fibrous, and
it seemed to have become interconnected with the metal
device. With time and determination, I removed all of my
flesh from the vessel. I boiled it for a while, aiming to sani-
tize it and remove any remaining organic material.

It was beautiful. The titanium vessel was shiny and flawless,
like highly polished silver. It proudly sported its company
brand name, Bard, like a Shakespearean call to tell a
story. The self-sealing, silicone rubber insertion site was a
rounded bubble that seemed to emit opaque light, almost
like a subdued gem. Visually speaking, it clearly appeared
as a charm or pendant of some sort, belying its nature as a
hidden, ideally inconspicuous, implant. I found a necklace
chain, polished it up to match, strung it with the medical
jewel, and wore it around my neck.

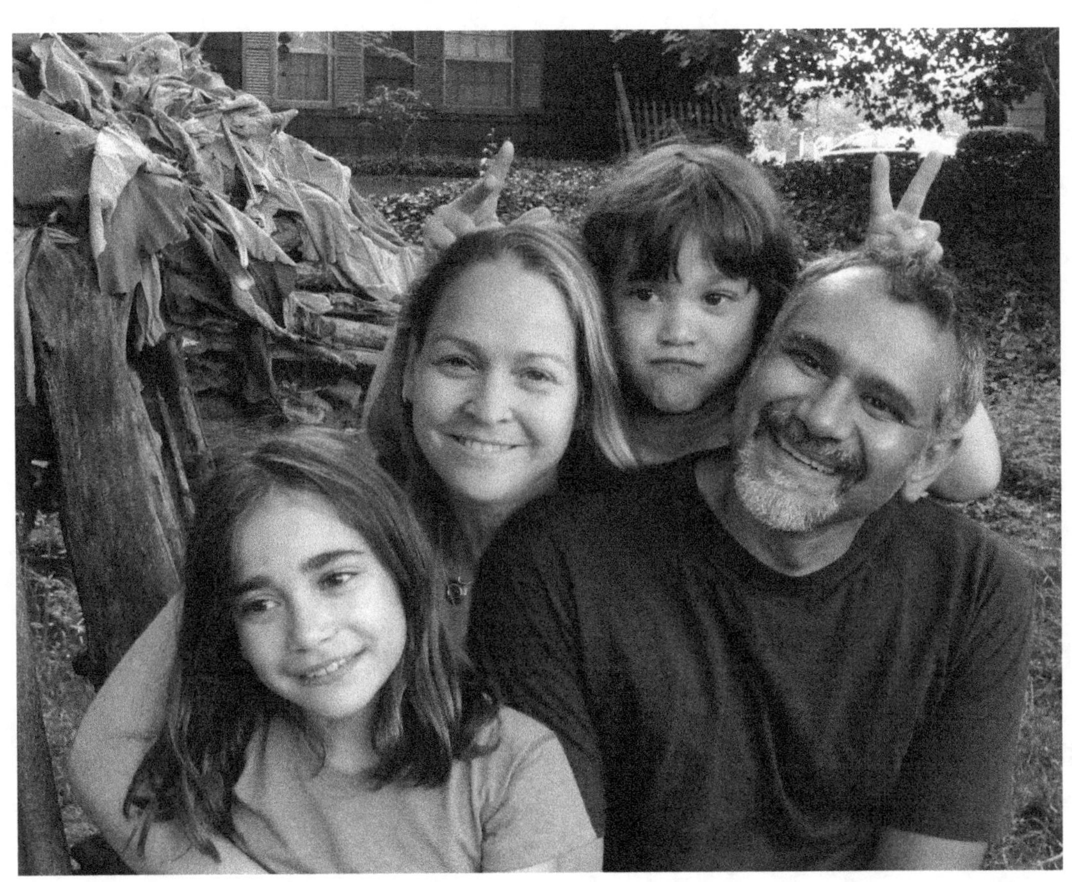

Lucy, Jessica, Kiran, and Amit
June 2013

Acknowledgements

Thank you to the mentors and colleagues who supported this
project: Ann Blackwell, Vicci Veenstra, Carol Jacobson, and Joanne
Leonard; Simon Gikandi, Anita Norich, and Ross Chambers;
Jonathan Schroeder, Therese Mulligan, Clarence Burton Sheffield,
Jr., Robert Ulin, Tina Lent, Carla Williams, Meredith Davenport,
Christine Shank, Angela Kelly, and Albert J. Winn.

Respect to the RIT Press team who recognized the value of
the story: Molly Q. Cort, Marnie Soom and David Pankow.
Appreciation to Elizabeth Lamark and Edgar Praus.

Love to friends who supported me, past and present:
Jeremy and Amy, Creighton, Colin and Wendy, Lee and Caroline,
Sylvia, Bradley, Jeff, Thomas, Jimmy, Kenny, Hal and Trey, Jen and
Lou, Jon and Elizabeth, Jordan and Jen, Ted, Victor, Lisa, Lara, Tim,
Linda, Richard and Danese, Babak and Jenny, Cathy and Larry,
Sandra, David, Toby, Kim, Eleanor, Wendy, Vicki, Hope, Shey, MG,
Laura, Kristin, Kim, Renee, Sheila, Chika, Ashley and Sarah.

Gratitude to those who made and make the difference:
Tina and Jim, Janelle and Charly, Sheri,
Emily and the Gerber family,
Mason and Rami, Donald and Patti, Rich and Ellen,
Ruth and Mitch, Fred and Effie,
Dr. HP and his team, Dr. EC, Lena, and Lucy Noll's Children's
Cancer Group.

To my family, who are all of the above:
Grandma Lucy,
Kevin, Freddy, Brandon,
Molly and Cory,
Erika and Barry,
Amit, Lucy and Kiran.

Appendix

Further Reading and Viewing in Visual Pathography

Batiuk, Tom. *Lisa's Story: The Other Shoe*. Kent, Ohio: Kent State University Press, 2007.

Blackburn, Amy. *Caring For Cynthia: A Caregiver's Journey through Breast Cancer*. Self-published, 2008.

Byram, Stephanie, Jennifer Matesa, and Charlee Brodsky. *Knowing Stephanie*. Pittsburgh: University of Pittsburgh Press, 2003.

Chronicle Books Staff. *Art. Rage. Us.: Art and Writing by Women with Breast Cancer*. San Francisco: Chronicle Books, 1998.

Coe, Sue. "AIDS." Graphic Witness. http://graphicwitness.org/coe/aids1.htm

Connolly, Harry, Tom Clancy, and Curt I. Civin. *Fighting Chance: Journeys through Childhood Cancer*. Baltimore: Woodholm House, 1998.

Creative Center. *Still Life: Documenting Cancer Survivorship*. New York: Umbrage Editions, 2007.

Davidson, Laura. *Voices from My Cancer Year*. Boston: Laura Davidson, 2005.

Davis, Amelia. *The First Look*. Urbana: University of Illinois Press, 2000.

Edson, Margaret. *W;t*. New York: Faber and Faber, Inc., 1993.

Fies, Brian. *Mom's Cancer*. Abrams ComicArts, 2006.

Freeheld. Film, 40 min. Directed by Cynthia Wade. U.S.: Lieutenant Films Inc., 2007.

Hunsicker, Jackson. *Turning Heads: Portraits of Grace, Inspiration, and Possibilities*. Sherman Oaks, CA: Press on Regardless, 2006.

I Photograph to Remember. CD-ROM, 35 min. Directed by Jonathan Green. New York: Voyager, 1991. http://www.pedromeyer.com/galleries/i-photograph/index.html.

Kandhola, Max. *Illustration of Life*. Syracuse, New York: Light Work, 2002.

Leibovitz, Annie. *A Photographer's Life: 1990-2005*. New York: Random House, 2006.

Lorant, Terry. *Reconstructing Aphrodite*. Syracuse, NY: Syracuse University Press, 2001.

Lynch, Dorothea, and Eugene Richards. *Exploding into Life*. New York: Aperture, 1986.

Mann, Sally. *Proud Flesh*. New York: Aperture/Gagosian Gallery, 2009.

Meyers, Art, and Maria Marrocchino. *Winged Victory: Altered Images: Transcending Breast Cancer*. San Diego: Photographic Gallery of Fine Art Books, 1996.

Meynell, Katharine, and Alistair Skinner. *It's Inside*. New York: Marion Boyars, 2005.

Murray, Lisa, and Billy Howard. *Angels and Monsters: A Child's Eye View of Cancer*. Atlanta, GA: American Cancer Society, 2002.

Neumayer, Leigh, Jay Agarwal, and Anne Vinsel. *Meet Virginia: Biography of a Breast*. Self-published, 2010.

Nikpay, Jila. *Heroines: Transformation in the Face of Breast Cancer*. Minneapolis: Zenith Services, 2006.

Photosensitive. *Cancer Connections: Images of Hope and Courage across Canada*. Mississauga, Ontario: John Wiley and Sons Canada Ltd., 2011.

Redgrave, Lynn, and Annabel Clark. *Journal: A Mother and Daughter's Recovery from Breast Cancer*. New York: Umbrage Editions.

Rosenthal, Ted. *How Could I Not Be Among You?* New York: Persea Books, 1973.

Springer, Melissa. *A Tribe of Warrior Women*. Birmingham: Crane Hill Publishers, 1996.

Tarr, Pam. *Journey: The Many Faces of Cancer*. Bloomington: AuthorHouse, 2007.

Terminals Project. http://vv.arts.ucla.edu/terminals/main.html.

Toledano, Phillip. *Days With My Father*. San Francisco: Chronicle Books, 2012. http://www.dayswithmyfather.com

Underhill, Linn. *Thirty Five Years/One Week*. Rochester: Visual Studies Workshop Press, 1981.

Further Reading and Viewing in Visual Autopathography

Adams, Ruth. "Unremarkable." Ruth Adams Photography, 2004.

Arneson, Robert. "Chemo Series." San Francisco Museum of Modern Art. http://www.sfmoma.org/explore/collection/artists/32/artwork.

Athey, Ron. Ronatheynews.blogspot.com.

Blue. Film, 79 min. Directed by Derek Jarman. London: Basilisk Communications, 1993.

"Christine Federighi." Clayscupture.com: Ceramics, Sculpture & Functional Art. http://infolinkmiami.com/cs/chrisf/chris.html.

"Christine Federighi: 2006 Fellow in Visual Arts 3D." Florida Division of Cultural Affairs. http://www.florida-arts.org/programs/fellowship/displayfellow.cfm?id=135.

Edwards, John D. *How Cancer Saved My Life.* Edited by Guy Bolam. London: BolamRose, 2013.

Farrah's Story. Documentary, 120 min. Directed by Alana Stewart. NBC, May 15, 2009.

Federighi, Christine. Ceramics, Sculpture & Functional Art: http://www.infolinkmiami.com/cs/chrisf/chris.html ClaySculpture.com.

———. Florida Division of Cultural Affairs: http://www.florida-arts.org/programs/fellowship/displayfellow.cfm?id=135.

Gonzalez-Torres, Felix, and Nancy Spector. *Felix Gonzalez-Torres.* Guggenheim Museum, 2007.

Guibert, Hervé. *La Pudeur ou L'impudeur.* 1991. Broadcast TF1, January 30, 1992.

Haring, Keith. The Keith Haring Foundation. Haring.com.

Kahlo, Frida, and Carlos Fuentes. *The Diary of Frida Kahlo: An Intimate Self-Portrait.* New York: Harry N. Abrams, Inc., 2005.

Kliman, Ted. "The Lamentation Series." Viewpoints-Zenith Gallery, 2008. http://www.zenithgallery.com/shows/2008/VIEWPOINTS%20Kliman.htm.

————. "Artery 717's Photos." MySpace page for Artery 717: http://www.myspace.com/artery717/photos/albums/ted-kliman/575008.

Lynn, Darcy. *Myself Resolved: An Artist's Experience With Lymphoma*. Philadelphia: Meniscus Ltd., 1994.

Lord, Catherine. *The Summer of Her Baldness: A Cancer Improvisation*. Austin, TX: University of Texas Press, 2004.

Loughridge, Sally. *Rad Art: A Journey through Radiation Treatment*. American Cancer Society, 2012.

Marchetto, Marisa Acocella. *Cancer Vixen*. New York: Knopf, 2006.

Pekar, Harvey, and Joyce Brabner. *Our Cancer Year*. Running Press, 1994.

Sick: The Life and Death of Bob Flanagan, Supermasochist. DVD, 90 min. Directed by Kirby Dick. Santa Monica, CA: Lion's Gate, 1997.

Silverlake Life: The View from Here. DVD, 99 min. Directed by Peter Friedman and Tom Joslin. New Media Group, 2003.

Spence, Jo. *Cultural Sniping: The Art of Transgression*. London: Routledge, 1995.

————. "A Picture of Health?" *Putting Myself in the Picture: A Political, Personal and Photographic Autobiography*. Seattle: Real Comet Press, 1988.

Utermohlen, William. www.williamutermohlen.org. Paris: Galerie Becket Odille Boicos, 2008-9.

Wilke, Hannah. *Intra Venus*. New York: Ronald Feldman Fine Arts, 1995.

Winn, Albert J. *Albert J. Winn Photographs*. 2010. Albertjwinn.com.

Wojnarowicz, David. *Memories that Smell Like Gasoline*. San Francisco: Artspace Books, 1992.

WORKS CITED

Aronson, Jeffrey, and Rachel Hall-Clifford. *The Patients' Tales Collection.* http://www.patientstales.org.

Barthes, Roland. 1981. *Camera Lucida: Reflections on Photography.* Translated by Richard Howard. New York: Farrar, Straus and Giroux.

Bennett, Jill. 2005. *Empathic Vision: Affect, Trauma, and Contemporary Art.* Stanford, CA: Stanford University Press.

Bjerke, Carol Chase. 2008. *Hidden Agenda.* Chicago: Borderland Books.

Butler, Judith. 2004. *Precarious Life: The Powers of Mourning and Violence.* Brooklyn, NY: Verso.

Caruth, Cathy. 1995. *Trauma: Explorations in Memory.* Baltimore: Johns Hopkins University Press.

Cazdyn, Eric. 2012. *The Already Dead.* Durham, NC: Duke University Press.

Couser, G. Thomas. 1997. *Recovering Bodies: Illness, Disability, and Life Writing.* Madison: University of Wisconsin.

Darts, David. 2012. "Opening 15X5 lightning talks: 'What is visual culture now?'" Paper presented at the Now! Visual Culture Conference, New York University, New York, May 31-June 2.

Frank, Arthur W. 1995. *The Wounded Storyteller: Body, Illness, and Ethics.* Chicago: University of Chicago Press.

Guibert, Hervé. 1991. *La Pudeur ou L'impudeur.* Broadcast TF1 January 30, 1992.

Hall, Martha A. *Holding In, Holding On: Artist's Books.* Northampton, MA: Mortimer Rare Book Room Publications, 2003.

Hunsaker Hawkins, Anne. 1999. *Reconstructing Illness: Studies in Pathography.* West Lafayette, Indiana: Purdue University Press.

120

Jarman, Derek. 1993. *Blue*. Film. Directed by Derek Jarman. UK: Basilisk Communications Ltd.

Joslin, Tom. 1993. *Silverlake Life: The View from Here*. Film. Directed by Peter Friedman and Tom Joslin. U.S.: New Video Group.

Lable, Eliot. 2006. *Intensity: The Milstein Series*. Long Island City, NY: Green/Lable.

Leibovitz, Annie. 2006. *A Photographer's Life: 1990-2005*. New York: Random House.

Lord, Catherine. 2004. *The Summer of Her Baldness: A Cancer Improvisation*. Austin, TX: University of Texas Press.

Loughridge, Sally. 2012. *Rad Art: A Journey Through Radiation Treatment*. Atlanta, GA: American Cancer Society.

Marchetto, Marisa Acocella. 2006. *Cancer Vixen*. New York: Knopf.

Marsted, Marcia Reid. 2002. *About My Hair: A Journey to Recovery*. Capelli d'Angeli.

Pekar, Harvey, and Joyce Brabner. 1994. *Our Cancer Year*. Philadelphia: Running Press.

Rosler, Martha. 2004. *Decoys and Disruptions: Selected Writings, 1975-2001*. Cambridge: MIT Press.

Saltzman, Lisa, and Eric Rosenberg. 2006. *Trauma and Visuality in Modernity*. Lebanon, NH: Dartmouth College Press.

Sontag, Susan. *Illness as Metaphor* (1978) *and AIDS and Its Metaphors*. 2001. New York: Picador.

———. 1977. *On Photography*. New York: Picador.

———. 2004a. *Regarding the Pain of Others*. New York: Picador.

———. "Regarding the Torture of Others." *The New York Times Magazine*, May 23, 2004b. Accessed May 17, 2013. http://www.nytimes.com/2004/05/23/magazine/regarding-the-torture-of-others. html?pagewanted=all&src=pm

Spence, Jo. 1988. *Putting Myself in the Picture: A Political, Personal, and Photographic Autobiography*. Seattle: Real Comet Press.

Squiers, Carol. 2005. *The Body at Risk: Photography of Disorder, Illness and Healing*. Berkeley: University of California Press and New York: International Center of Photography.

Taylor, Diana. 2012. "Opening 15×5 lightning talks: 'What is visual culture now?'" Paper presented at the Now! Visual Culture Conference, New York University, New York, May 31-June 2, 2012.

Toombs, S. Kay. 1992. *The Meaning of Illness: A Phenomenological Account of the Different Perspectives of Physician and Patient*. Norwell, MA: Kluwer Academic Publishers.

Wilke, Hannah. 1995. *Intra Venus*. New York: Ronald Feldman Fine Arts, Inc.

———. 1998. *Hannah Wilke: A Retrospective*. Copenhagen: Nicolaj, Copenhagen Contemporary Art Center. Elisabeth Hansen, ed.

Winn, Albert J. 2010. *Albert J. Winn Photographs*. Albertjwinn.com.

Wojnarowicz, David. *PPOW Gallery*. Accessed May 20, 2012
http://www.ppowgallery.com/selected_work.php?artist=14

Zylinska, Joanna. 2012. "Interdisciplinarity." Paper presented at the Now! Visual Culture Conference, New York University, New York, May 31-June 2, 2012.

LIST OF ILLUSTRATIONS

Colophon

Designed by Marnie Soom

Typeset in Scala

Printed by Lightning Source

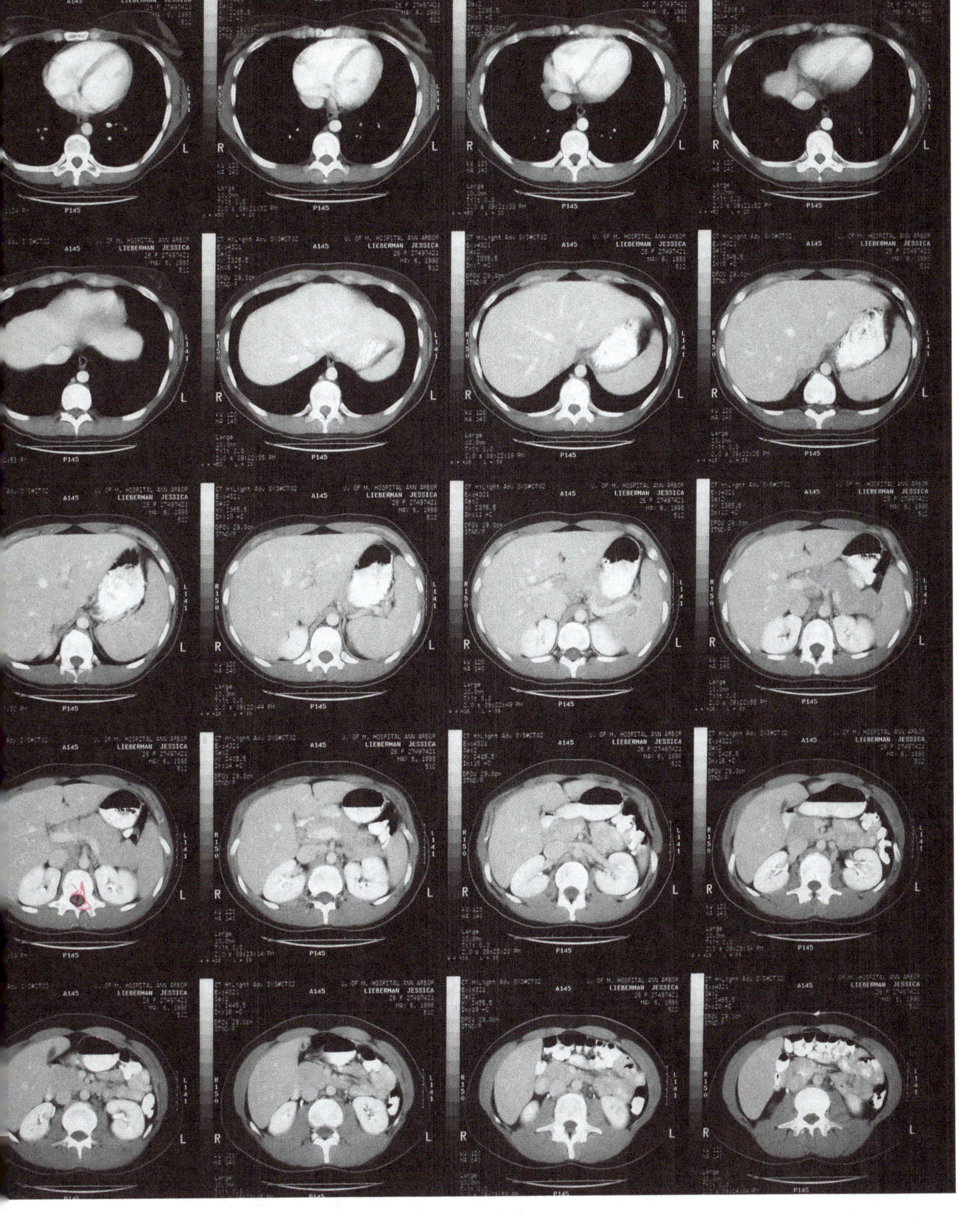

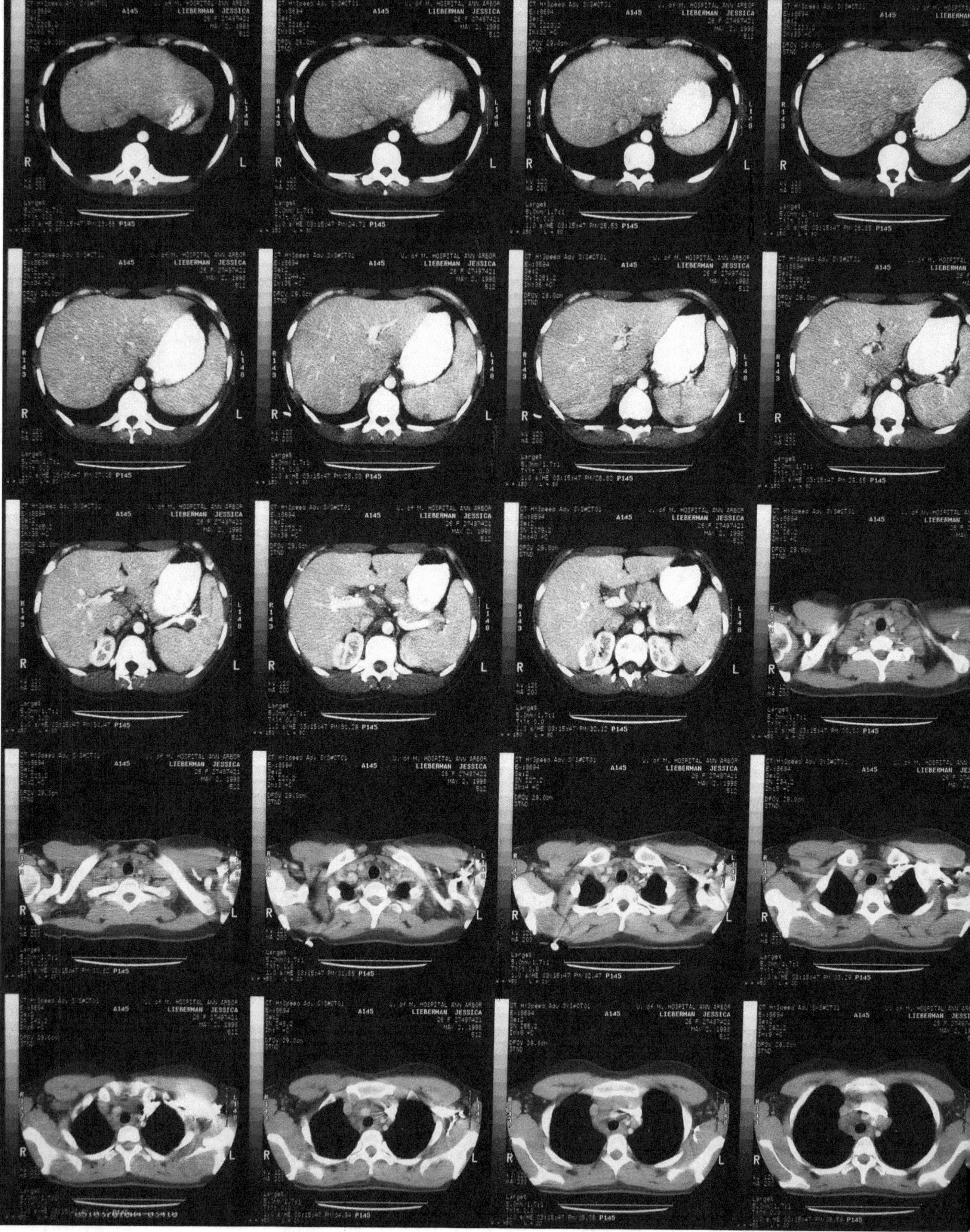

www.ingramcontent.com/pod-product-compliance
Lightning Source LLC
Chambersburg PA
CBHW081415250726
48654CB00013B/1710